Care Work, Migrant Peasant Families and Discourse of Filial Piety in China

Longtao He

Care Work, Migrant Peasant Families and Discourse of Filial Piety in China

palgrave
macmillan

Longtao He
Research Institute of Social Development
Southwestern University of Finance and Economics
Chengdu, China

The proofreading of the final book manuscript was partially funded by MOE (Ministry of Education in China) Youth Project of Humanities and Social Sciences (project No.: 20XJC840001). This funder has no role in the research design, the writing of the article, or the decision to submit the article.

ISBN 978-981-16-1879-6 ISBN 978-981-16-1880-2 (eBook)
https://doi.org/10.1007/978-981-16-1880-2

This Palgrave Macmillan imprint is published by the registered company Springer Nature Singapore Pte Ltd.
The registered company address is: 152 Beach Road, #21-01/04 Gateway East, Singapore 189721, Singapore

Foreword

In this book, Associate Professor Longtao He explores complex reflections on caregiving and filial piety, narrated by 24 Chinese migrant workers who have returned from the big cities in which they have been working to look after parents with terminal illnesses. My relationship with the author started as a Ph.D. supervisor and continues as a colleague, but in many ways I was also a student who was privileged to join this research journey. He, himself originally from the rural and significantly cancer-affected province of Sichuan in which the research took place, undertook a culturally localised Foucauldian discourse analysis of interviews and observations that took place in a local hospital. The analysis of data simultaneously and carefully balanced and navigated concepts drawn from western methodology and from an action/practice orientation (mainly Confucian) that was grounded in 'Chineseness'. International readers will encounter a treasure trove of personal and professional academic insights. Those insights include not only the methodological innovations that were crafted but also revelations of how Chinese migrant workers experience caregiving, how filial piety is both a burden and a precious intergenerational resource, and how practical and policy-related challenges require articulation and recognition so that they might be overcome. The text is relevant well beyond the domain of China as its contents will enlighten western-based health researchers, practitioners, and policymakers seeking to understand diverse cultural perspectives.

Kate van Heugten
Professor
School of Language, Social and Political Sciences
University of Canterbury
Christchurch, New Zealand

Acknowledgements

This book grew out of my Ph.D. thesis. I could not have completed it without the gracious help and support of many people.

First of all, I am overwhelmingly grateful to Professor Kate van Heugten, my senior supervisor for my Ph.D. at the University of Canterbury in New Zealand and a generous colleague since my graduation in 2018. Her comprehensive knowledge of the human services discipline and social sciences in general has helped me in every step of my thesis writing and in the preparation of post-thesis publications. She has been extremely supportive and kind through the life difficulties I encountered both during and after the Ph.D. programme. I could not have written this book without her help and guidance.

I would like to thank my parents, Junfang He 何俊芳 and Haiyang He 何海洋, who have always been my rock, and my two-year-old son, Xuanhan He 何轩翰 (the sunshine of my life); my friends Chia-Chen Pan (潘家甄), Misato Makino, and Jasper Obico; my colleagues Dr. Zhifang Song, Dr. Maria Perez-Y-Perez, Prof. Jianbin Xu (许建斌), Prof. Wenjie Duan (段文杰), and Prof. Huamin Peng (彭华民); my student, Furong Shi (师芙蓉); my copyeditor, Mona-Lynn Courteau; and my Ph.D. colleagues Dr. Chandan Bose, Lu Zhou (周璐), Anmeng Liu (刘安盟), and Dr. Tuhina Varghese for their friendship and support during the writing of the book manuscript.

Contents

About the Author

Longtao He is a Health & Medical Sociologist and an Associate Professor in the Research Institute of Social Development at Southwestern University of Finance and Economics, Chengdu, China. His research interests and expertise include: qualitative methodologies (especially Foucauldian discourse analysis) for health & medical sociology, qualitative studies in mental health and health psychology, ethics studies in public health and social work, informal caregiver issues in relation to eldercare in China. He has published numerous articles in SSCI/SCI journals, such as *Qualitative Health Research, British Journal of Social Work, BMJ Open, European Journal of Ageing*, and so on.

CHAPTER 1

The Care Burden of Chinese Migrant Peasant Workers

Introduction

> It is only *tianjingdiyi* [natural] to take care of your own parents. Human beings have to be filial. (P1: a daughter, aged 41–50, remarried, father was ill)

> The pattern of filial piety is nearly the same in our generation, my parents' generation, and the ones before. However, my children's generation might not be the same. Money has outweighed almost everything, including morals, in China today. Filial piety is not regarded to be as important as it was before. (P2: a daughter, aged 31–40, married, father was ill)

The above comments were made by two migrant peasant workers whose fathers had each been diagnosed with cancer a few months earlier. Participant 1 (P1)'s comment reflects the close and overlapping relationship in China between the provision of caregiving to parents and filial piety. Filial piety refers to a Chinese cultural norm that requires children to provide care, to respect, and to show obedience to their parents (see Terry et al. [2016] for a discussion of filial piety in the twenty-first century). Filial piety is one of the most profound values that govern family relationships across all Confucian cultural societies. Filial piety regulates the rights and obligations between parents and children, facilitates interactions between generations, and enhances social cohesion and integration

L. He, *Care Work, Migrant Peasant Families and Discourse of Filial Piety in China*, https://doi.org/10.1007/978-981-16-1880-2_1

(Chan et al., 2012). Empirical research has examined the role that filial piety plays in the motivations for family caregiving and has investigated factors influencing the well-being of caregivers (Chan et al., 2012).

According to P1, taking care of one's parents is a way of being filial, and filial piety is a responsibility that human beings must fulfil. P2's comment reflects the status quo of the Chinese welfare system. The Chinese welfare system for elders, especially rural elders, is not as developed and comprehensive as the welfare systems that exist in some western countries. For P2, it seemed as though the notion of filial piety had not changed for centuries, and yet she thought that future generations might not be as filial as preceding generations. In her explanation, P2 thought that the rise of consumerism and the valorisation of money was at the root of a degradation in filial piety. This view may reflect a romanticised nostalgia about the past and fears about the consequences of current changes with respect to filial practices and perceptions.

This book aims to discover how Chinese migrant peasant workers, such as the two participants mentioned above, view their care experiences for their ill parents. Filial piety is a fundamental concept and responsibility for Chinese people as human beings, as noted by P1, and can therefore be expected to play an important role in how people make sense of their care practices, experiences, and perceptions. I adopted a discursive perspective in order to examine the mechanisms and content of the discourses that pertain to filial care, and in particular how those discourses shaped participants' care experiences. In an ever-changing China, traditional values and practices are facing enormous challenges through contextual alterations such as rapid and massive urbanisation, globalisation, and the prevalence of public education (Lin, 2013; Rofel, 2007; Wang, 2016). The fear that future generations will not be as filial attracts the interest not only of people who are caring for older persons but also of policymakers and academics who attempt to make sense of how filial piety is constructed socially in the present, and what various political, social, economic, and/or cultural contexts will be likely to impact on this construct in the immediate and longer term future.

In China since the 1978 economic reform, social, economic, and political changes have been taking place that have given rise to increasing care needs of elder cancer patients, and concomitantly to increasing care burdens of their adult children. This is particularly so for migrant peasant workers, that is, people who have migrated back and forth from rural areas to coastal or other cities within China with booming economies and job opportunities, often to work in blue-collar factory jobs or in low-level positions in small private companies and always remaining in a state of migration/temporariness. There is a trend towards diminishing informal care practices and filial piety in contemporary Chinese society, and this appears especially true in terms of the filial care practices of migrant peasant workers. This chapter focuses on how these socio-economic changes might be affecting migrant peasant workers' care burdens.

Increasing Need for Care of Elderly Cancer Patients in China

Since the 1990s, China has been experiencing both extremely fast population ageing and increasing incidences of various cancers (Chen, 2009; Chen et al., 2016). These have inevitably led to increased care needs of elder cancer patients in China. After nearly 30 years of economic reforms and rapid economic growth, China's demographic profile demonstrates two clear trends: significant ageing of the population and a dropping fertility rate (Zhang et al., 2012). According to Yi and George (2010) and Zeng et al. (2013), the average life expectancy in China increased to 73 years in 2005, a marked increase from 41 years in 1950, the year after the founding of the People's Republic of China. Zeng et al. (2013) estimate that the average life expectancy for both sexes will reach 84.8 years by 2050. At the same time, fertility rates have declined dramatically, to between 1.6 and 1.8 children per woman in 2005, from the 1950s when the birth rate exceeded six children per woman (Zeng et al., 2013).

According to many scholars, the reduction in family size is also largely due to the success of the one-child policy (Hesketh et al., 2005; Wang et al., 2005). The one-child policy, implemented in 1979, ruled that a married couple was only allowed to have one child (Hesketh et al., 2005). Some scholars (e.g., Cai, 2010) have suggested that the one-child policy might not be the real cause of the drop in fertility rate; others (Feng et al., 2013) acknowledge other factors—such as urbanisation, fear of famine (1959–1961), social changes caused by the Great Leap Forward (in the 1950s), the collectivisation campaign of the 1950s, and the Cultural Revolution (1966–1976)—but maintain that the one-child policy remains a major contributor to China's fertility rate falling below the replacement rate. There are many factors in the drop in fertility, such as the prevalence of individualism, the rise of women's rights, and the increasing divorce rate. Another important factor is high pressure from an economic perspective to raise children in contemporary China according to microeconomic theory (Wang et al., 2011). In 2000, 6.7% of the Chinese population was over 65-years old (Gallagher-Thompson et al., 2012). However, even on the basis of a high mortality rate assumption, the cohort of 65-year-olds and older is expected to constitute more than 24% of the population in China by 2050 (Gallagher-Thompson et al., 2012).

While ageing is a complicated phenomenon that depends on the interaction between genetics, behaviour, and physiology, and considering that the effect of prolonged longevity is difficult to predict, the connection between advanced age and the prevalence of health problems is well established on an individual level (Zimmer, 2016). According to Tang et al. (2013), the incidence rate of cancer cases has vastly increased in China in recent years, and it has become the leading cause of death there. Chen et al. (2016) identify particular attributes of cancer in China: that lung cancer has become the leading cause of cancer death, followed by oesophageal, stomach, and liver cancer; and that rural residents tend to have higher mortality rates than their urban counterparts for all types of cancers.

The increase in cancer rates in China in recent decades (Liu, 2004) can be attributed to numerous factors such as an ageing population, industrial pollution, and malnutrition (Blot et al., 1993; Gong et al., 2012; Xu et al., 1989). This heightens the urgency for developing improved care provision for older persons with cancer and for endeavouring to ensure they have a good quality of life towards the end of their lives (Phillips et al., 2010).

Informal Care

Increasing population ageing and cancer incidence highlight not only issues in relation to older cancer patients' quality of life but also the care burden for caregivers and their health status issues. In recent end-of-life care research, scholars have begun to recognise informal care as a crucial element in a holistic approach to achieving the well-being of people with advanced illness (Cohen & Deliens, 2012). The majority of people suffering from a serious illness cannot manage their care on their own and instead rely on family, friends, and the community (Papastavrou et al., 2009). According to the World Health Organization (n.d.-a, para. 1), '[p]alliative care is an approach that improves the quality of life of patients and their families facing the problem associated with life-threatening illness'. Policies for the promotion of palliative care aim to improve the quality of life for patients and to take into account the needs of their families, since family members usually also play the role of caregiver (Cohen et al., 2015). According to Applebaum and Breitbart (2013), comprehensive palliative care involves paying attention to the needs of patients as well as to those of their informal caregivers in order to address the need for both efficiency and effectiveness in ensuring patients' quality of life.

Hooyman and Kiyak (2008) concluded that many studies do not clearly define 'informal caregiver'. According to a literature review of informal caregiving articles spanning 10 years from 2000 until 2011 and mainly focused in the United Kingdom and the United States, 56% of articles did not define the term at all, and 12% narrowed it down for the purpose of their research to include only care given by family members such as a spouse or children (Aoun et al., 2013). Palm (2013) defined the term informal caregivers more broadly, to refer to those people who are not medical or other employed staff. From this perspective informal caregivers can include family members, relatives, friends, neighbours, and volunteer caregivers who provide assistance in patients' daily living, emotional support, medical assistance, funding, and so on. Informal caregiving is equated to that provided by family even though it includes more than just family members (Hooyman & Kiyak, 2008).

Among all the possible informal caregivers mentioned by Lin et al. (2020), adult children have an above-average responsibility for satisfying their elderly parents' needs. According to Palm (2013), the relationship between children and parents is a special kind of relationship that differs from companionship and friendship, and has a higher intrinsic value. Besides their spouses, ill parents are most vulnerable to their adult children because those children are in a unique position to fulfil their needs (Li et al., 2019). In the Chinese context, adult children are accorded a special moral responsibility, rooted in filial piety, to support and care for their parents. While recognising that informal caregivers can include other family members and friends, for the purpose of my research, participating informal caregivers included only adult children and daughters-in-law (considering the important care role the daughter-in-law plays in traditional China; Palm, 2013).

According to Pizzo et al. (2015), informal caregivers act as both care coordinators and service providers and contribute tremendously to patients' well-being. According to Palm (2013), it is more likely for elderly parents who are cared for by their children to also gain access to formal care than it is for those parents without such support, since children often assist with applications for formal care. Informal caregivers experience an increased or decreased sense of burden depending on the level of the patient's pain and psychological distress. The increases or decreases in the well-being of the informal caregiver also correlate with the patient's quality of life (Contro et al., 2002).

In addition, lack of sufficient and affordable social institutions for eldercare increases the importance of informal caregivers. In China, a number of policies have been aimed at building up the eldercare service system. These policies still mainly rely on home care (PRWeb, 2013). Many cities in China have proposed the '9073' plan which aims to ensure that '90% of elderly people with illness receive home-based care, 7% community-based care, and 3% institution-based care' (Albany, 2013, p. 4). However, the infrastructure for the 3% institutionalised care has not been put in place (Albany, 2013). Currently, only 1.2% of the older population are cared for in institutions compared to 8% in some western countries (Gallagher-Thompson et al., 2012). In addition to the low availability of institutionalised care, the cost of enrolling in Chinese public nursing homes has increased to an unaffordable level for most older Chinese people (Liu et al., 2019; Zhang et al., 2012).

There appears to be an increasing worry among rural older persons about the availability of care from their migrant peasant worker children. Most older persons with terminal diseases in China remain at home, which means they have to rely on informal care rather than formal and institutionalised care (Albany, 2013; Diamond, 2009). However, in recent years in rural China, elders have faced a low availability of caregivers due to adult children's migration for work (Wu et al., 2008; Zhang, 2019). Even though there is an urgent need for institutionalised care in rural areas, and although the Chinese government is trying to build more institutions for rural eldercare, Zhang (2019) strongly predicted that informal family care will remain the main source of care for rural elders in the foreseeable future. According to a study by Shi and Hu (2020), rural residents prefer family care as compared to institutionalised care. However, family care is strongly focused on care by a child, and there is a major concern that no child will be available to take care of them. In addition, older rural persons are also concerned about the cost of paying for their health care and basic living needs (Huang, 2018).

The participants in my research were members of a Chinese population cohort that had been significantly influenced by the latest economic reforms that started in 1979. Since 1979, China has opened its market to the outside world and shifted from a state-controlled economy to a market-oriented economy (Zhang & Shunfeng, 2003). This has led to a marked acceleration of urbanisation. People, mostly young, poured into big cities from rural areas (Chang, 1994; Zhu, 2001). This group of migrants is known as *min gong* (民工) or *nong min gong* (农民工), translated as migrant peasant workers by scholars such as Ngai and Huilin (2010). More than three decades into economic reforms, the parents of migrant peasant workers have grown old and remain living in the rural areas (Wang, 2016). In undertaking my research, I was interested to discover how family care is performed and practised by migrant peasant workers, particularly in the presence of advanced cancer.

Migrant peasant workers, compared to urban residents, are usually less privileged in terms of income and social status (Wong et al., 2007). According to Lin (2013), they are considered to be less modern and progressive by the general public. Lin's (2013) research revealed that male migrant peasant workers use filial piety as a means of making sense of themselves and their identity in the unfamiliar and unequal environments they encounter in the big cities in which they work. However, working and living in the city presents difficulties when it comes to taking care of their rural elderly parents in need, owing to the distances involved and the migrants' disadvantaged financial status (Joseph & Phillips, 1999). In addition, in the current market-oriented metropolitan cities, it is extremely difficult for migrant peasant workers to ask for leave, even unpaid leave, to visit their rural hometown to take care of parents in need (Lin, 2013). In addition to the lesser social status of migrant peasant workers in the metropolitan cities, rural families are also disadvantaged in terms of their access to social welfare provisions. This is discussed in the next section.

Insufficient Welfare System Provisions for Rural Families

Throughout Chinese history, arrangements for even the most basic welfare have been rooted in and have relied on the provision of family support (Gruijters, 2017). In comparison with western countries, family care is significantly more prevalent than institutional care for older persons in China (Jackson & Liu, 2017). Regardless of the government's more recent attention to the need for improved support, China has not built up a very comprehensive social security system for older persons, especially those living in rural areas (Liu & Sun, 2016). This lack of sufficient welfare provisions results in family usually being the main, and often only, resource for end-of-life care. The rising cost of health care and expanding long-term disease patterns in recent decades (Burns & Liu, 2017) has furthermore led to the financial burden on patients and family caregivers becoming ever more challenging.

Pension Schemes

After the economic reforms, the bankruptcy and downsizing of many state-owned enterprises created sustainability issues for the former *danwei* (单位, government department or state-owned enterprise) based urban pension system (Liu & Sun, 2016). The collapse of the rural commune system destroyed financial support for older persons living in rural areas (Williamson et al., 2012). Instead, a multi-pillar system has been introduced, which covers three state-funded pension programmes. The first is the pension programme for government and public-sector workers. This is thought to be the best social security programme, but it only covered 5% of the workforce in the year 2008 (Williamson et al., 2012). The second, the urban pension system, also called Basic Old-Age Insurance, covered 28% of the total workforce, while the third, the voluntary rural pension scheme, covered 7% of the total workforce (Williamson et al., 2012). There is a huge gap between the provisions of these three schemes (Salditt et al., 2007). The first programme offered the best terms for beneficiaries (Salditt et al., 2007). I will focus on the last programme, the rural pension scheme, since that is relevant for my research.

According to Liu and Sun (2016), the Chinese government has been trying to expand the coverage of and reduce the gap between these three schemes. In 2009, a new rural pension scheme was piloted in a few counties (Gao et al., 2012), after which the programme was rolled out. The new rural pension scheme contains two tiers: (1) a voluntary funded defined contribution component and (2) a non-contributory social pension component (Williamson et al., 2017). If an adult child joins the scheme voluntarily, both parents receive a 70 RMB (approximately 10 USD) social pension irrespective of whether they themselves have joined the scheme (Williamson et al., 2017). For the funded defined contribution tier, participants in the scheme choose to pay between 100 RMB and 2,000 RMB per year (around 15–290 USD) for more than 15 years. According to H. Ma (2015), the average yearly income in rural Sichuan province (where I carried out my fieldwork) was around 7,000 RMB (1,000 USD). Once the participants reach the age of eligibility, they receive a pension allowance relative to the level of their payment. Men become eligible to receive the pension when they reach the age of 60 years and women when they reach the age of 55 (Williamson et al., 2017).

In 2008, there were a number of small schemes in place that together only covered 10% of rural residents (Williamson et al., 2017). According to Williamson et al. (2017), by the end of 2014, most rural residents who were over the threshold age were eligible to join the new rural pension scheme. The scheme later expanded to unemployed urban residents and other urban social groups such as homemakers (Gao et al., 2012). According to Williamson et al. (2017), the gap between the urban pension and the rural pension has been narrowed owing to the Chinese government's efforts. For example, the fully state-funded pension system for government and public-sector servants was abolished in 2014 (Liu & Sun, 2016). After the abolition, public servants became subject to the less lucrative urban employee social pension schemes.

Liu and Sun (2016) claimed that suggestions that provisions made under the rural pension scheme have expanded are exaggerated. They also explained that the average allowance (80 RMB/12 USD per month) is too small to cover daily living costs. (To put this into perspective, according to Williamson et al. (2012), 1 kg of pork cost more than 30 RMB in 2012.) Moreover, although eligible, people in rural areas, and especially young people with parents in rural areas, are reluctant to join the new rural pension scheme (Liu & Sun, 2016). Only four out of my 24 participants had joined the pension scheme (one of them had joined the urban employee pension scheme). No participants' parents joined the voluntary tier of the new rural pension scheme. According to Gao et al. (2012), there is concern about the trustworthiness and reliability of the programme, since the pension accounts are not transparent and the funding financed by individual accounts is mainly used to cover current beneficiaries. Thus, many migrant peasant workers refuse to participate in the new rural pension scheme. In the meantime, most employers still refuse to include migrant workers in workplace-based pension programmes, despite the government's efforts to promote the welfare of migrant peasant workers in private companies and factories (OECD, 2012).

Social and Health Insurance in Rural China

Although health insurance schemes have been relatively successful in terms of achieving national coverage, funding for these schemes remains insufficient. Since the initiation of the New Rural Cooperative Medical Scheme in 2003, its coverage has extended to 833,000,000 rural residents, including migrant peasant workers, accounting for nearly 90% of the rural population (Babiarz et al., 2010). (Migrant peasant workers are considered to be rural 'residents' because their registrations are still rural, even though they work and live in urban areas.) In order to control the financial risk, China's medical insurance schemes greatly depend on high co-payments (the part that the patient needs to pay each time a medical service is accessed), which means that services are often unaffordable for rural residents (Li et al., 2012). In recent years, China's rural medical insurance schemes have been specifically designed to protect against catastrophic diseases such as cancer, and episodes of major illness and hospitalisation (Blumenthal & Hsiao, 2015; Social Security Official Website, 2017). According to the Social Security Official Website (2017), several cancers including stomach, oesophageal, colon, and rectal cancer have reached reimbursement rates as high as 80% in many regions.

Despite this, however, out of pocket expenses for the insured rural families are still too high (Xing, 2015). Long-term care for someone suffering from a chronic condition is not included in the coverage (Xing, 2015). Outpatient services, rehabilitation, routine essential drugs, and hospice care (care aimed at alleviating pain for patients with terminal illness and to fulfil their last wishes) are not prioritised by these schemes (Li et al., 2012). Langzhong city, where I undertook my fieldwork, initiated a special social insurance policy to aid people suffering catastrophic diseases (in association with the New Rural Cooperative Medical Scheme which varies from region to region). Catastrophic diseases that are covered under the policy include stomach and oesophageal cancer (the main types of cancer with which my participants' parents had been diagnosed). The policy covered up to 75–80% of most of the inpatient expenditures. However, limited or no coverage is provided for many necessary medicines, nutrition fluids, bed fees for family caregivers, outpatient services, and so on (Zhang et al., 2010).

Other Governmental Support Policies

The way in which the new rural pension enables children to purchase cover for their parents can be seen as a form of governmental support for caregivers and their families. It also reinforces the notion that family members are responsible for one another, binding them together. However, considering the extremely limited coverage of the new rural pension discussed above, such governmental support for caregivers is minimal.

There are other approaches to incentivising family caregiving, such as the inheritance law that favours children fulfilling filial obligations with rights to inherit a larger portion of their deceased parents' estate (Chou, 2011). However, for many rural families, the promise of an inheritance may not provide sufficient incentive for a child to enter into a care agreement (Chou, 2011). Older persons in rural China are not often able to leave their children a large inheritance at this late stage of their life (Mao, 2010). Moreover, the law has not been specific about how parents should distribute family estates among children, or how to measure the fulfilment of filial obligations (Palm, 2013). Additionally, this law is unlikely to be effective in promoting family care in one-child families because there is only one child to inherit the family estate in any case.

There have been some sporadic improvements in policies for the support of home-based care for older persons that may offer some indirect support for family caregivers in some cities. For example, in cities such as Beijing and Shanghai, a few charitable organisations or the local government that provide small stipends and other forms of support to older persons with a catastrophic illness (such as cancer) and caregiving training to family members (Hu et al., 2020; Mao, 2010). However, overall there is still a significant lack of governmental support for informal caregivers (He & van Heugten, 2020; Mao, 2010). The need for such support is a long-standing international issue; for example, Barusch (1995) expressed her concern that in many countries lack of government support jeopardises family caregivers' investments in caring for their elders. In the next section, we will look at various forms of care burdens family caregivers might need to face, especially due to the lack of sufficient public support.

The Burden of Care for Informal Caregivers

The literature reflects increasing awareness of the burdens that informal caregivers bear when providing care for loved ones (Seo & Park, 2019; Xiao et al., 2014). In this section, I will briefly introduce the financial burdens, physical and emotional burdens, and cultural and philosophical burdens.

The insufficiency of pension and health insurance policies has resulted in a financial plight that both patients and informal caregivers, namely adult children, have to face (Jung & Liu Streeter, 2015). Out of pocket health expenditure (the part the patient's family has to pay) per capita has risen dramatically over the last 30 years in China. According to a review report on the Chinese health system from the World Health Organization in 2015, China showed a rapid growth rate in total health expenditure from 2005 to 2012. Although governmental health funding has increased greatly, the private and out of pocket health expenditure also peaked (World Health Organization, 2015).

Although there is no specific data on the percentage of out of pocket health expenditure covered by family caregivers, the above data can be used as a basis for the estimation of the financial burden for families. Even with the New Rural Cooperative Health Scheme and the special catastrophic disease protection policy associated with the scheme, there is still a popular saying among Chinese people: *Xinxinkuku 30 nian, yi bing hui dao jie fang qian* (辛辛苦苦三十年, 一病回到解放, once one becomes ill, one's savings amassed over 30 years of hard work will be depleted) (Xing, 2015, p. 14).

According to data from a 2010 study of family caregivers of cancer patients in China, 66.8% of caregivers made major life changes or gave up their job in order to provide care, 55% of families lost their main source of income, and 68% of families spent most of their savings on treatment and other related expenses (Lu et al., 2010). Moreover, informal caregivers, who have been seen as the 'invisible workforce', are often unpaid and unsupported (Meier, 2012). According to Meng (2013), providing informal care for ill family members has negative impacts in terms of reducing the paid hours of work for men by 48 minutes per 10 hours of care provided per week, and by 35 minutes per 10 hours of care provided by women.

In the Chinese context, hospitals do not provide sufficient bedside care for patients. Except for injections and fluid transmission, which are undertaken by nurses, care is provided by family members (Pan & Feng, 2007). That is to say, at least one member is required to remain in the hospital with the patient to provide everyday care such as feeding and washing the patient. According to Xu et al. (2016), the ratio of nurses and other professional caregivers per patient bed is far below that of western countries. In a study of nurses' absence in a Chinese hospital, Wang et al. (2014) suggested that research data for nurse-to-bed ratios rarely takes into account nurses' absences, which means the real situation with respect to the lack of professional hospital caregivers is likely to be even worse than the research shows.

In the field, I witnessed how busy the nurses were on a daily basis, and that a mere five or six nurses cared for patients in a department of approximately 45 beds. They had no time to provide patient care other than to give injections and set up fluid transmissions (besides their role of assisting the doctors and completing administrative tasks). Ultimately, many tasks such as the monitoring of fluid transmission and medical machine index changes, feeding, toileting, hospital paperwork processing, bathing, and so on, had to be undertaken by family members. Being available to undertake these tasks required family members to give up at least some of their paid working hours, and frequently they had no alternative but to completely cease work since, they struggled to obtain even unpaid leave (Ye et al., 2013). This loss of income significantly added to other financial burdens of the informal caregivers.

In order to assist older family members to have a 'good death', substantial support needs to be provided, which takes a physical and emotional toll on family members in addition to the economic costs they carry (Lu et al., 2010). Caregivers often experience anxiety and depression, sleep deprivation, social isolation, financial stress, and reduced quality of life, among other negative impacts (Ugalde et al., 2012). As a result, informal caregivers often report poorer health than non-caregivers (Rehman et al., 2009). Firstly, studies have shown that caregivers often express concerns about their physical health including fatigue or exhaustion, insomnia, and interrupted sleep (Aoun et al., 2013; Rehman et al., 2009). They may have difficulties caring for themselves due to lack of time. Secondly, caring for dying parents while attempting to maintain their own quality of life, renegotiating social roles and relationships, and dealing with emotional conflicts complicates caregivers' self-identity and their interactions with the patients and others in their social world (Ugalde et al., 2012). The factors discussed above might jeopardise caregivers' psychosocial health and cause mental and social problems such as depression, anxiety, and loss of informal and formal social relationships (Aoun et al., 2013).

According to a study undertaken by Liu et al. (2015), a majority of Chinese migrant peasant workers are susceptible to some kind of non-communicable disease because of the nature of their work, and their health status may therefore already be poorer than that of the general population. Another Chinese scholar, Mao (2010), claimed that informal caregivers who are older or in poor physical health are likely to carry a heavier care burden and incur more stress. As informal caregivers for their parents, they might also encounter conflicting roles as children, spouses, and even grandparents (Mao, 2010).

For many advanced cancer patients, death is considered a medical certainty in the intermediate term, if not imminent. Nonetheless, talking about death is not easy (Kortes-Miller, 2015). In western end-of-life care professions, many practitioners struggle to engage in open discussions about death with their patients, although it is a common practice to disclose the approaching death to patients (Kortes-Miller, 2015; Tse et al., 2003). Professional advisors may assess patients' symptoms and needs, ask about their wishes, and endeavour to enable patients to be involved in decision-making about future plans (Kortes-Miller, 2015).

In China, however, it is unusual for doctors and nurses to talk about death with terminal patients (Fang et al., 2009; Kendall, 2006). As a matter of fact, the truth about a patient's condition will most often not be revealed to the patient (Jiang et al., 2007). Instead of involving the patients themselves, adult children or spouses are normally asked to sign the surgery consent form if a surgery is needed or recommended by the doctor (Cong, 2004; Hancock et al., 2007). By not revealing the truth to parents, however, a family caregiver may suffer emotional distress and experience a sense of isolation in knowing the prognosis (Aoun et al., 2015; Tse et al., 2003). Keeping the prognosis secret prevents family members from seeking closure, for example by seeking or providing forgiveness for past deeds, expressing gratitude, or saying goodbye to their parents. The practice of not telling is also related to the cultural norm of filial piety, as talking about death to one's parents is often considered to be a taboo in filial discourses (Yick & Gupta, 2002).

Filial piety might also be a hindrance for building a welfare system for older persons. In several western countries, contributions made by unpaid informal carers have begun to be recognised by policymakers (Corden & Hirst, 2011). For instance, the United Kingdom government offers a small stipend, as well as retirement contributions, to family carers. A policy introduced by New Zealand Ministry of Health, effective from 2013, enabled disabled people to pay a family member for their caregiving activities (Disability Support Services, 2018). However, in large part due to the strongly held cultural norm of filial piety which assumes that care of older persons with advanced illnesses will be provided primarily (perhaps exclusively) by the family instead of by the government, it is common for families to take full responsibility for taking care of elderly parents in China (Gallagher-Thompson et al., 2012). Family caregivers (mainly referring to adult children in my research) rarely reach outside the family for help, due to strong filial piety and family values (Gallagher-Thompson et al., 2012).

From the above discussion, filial piety can be seen to constitute a cultural and philosophical 'burden' for children as caregivers. Patterson et al. (1998) argued, however, that caregiving does not necessarily undermine adult children's quality of life. According to the World Health Organization (n.d.-b, para. 2), quality of life is 'an individual's perception of their position in life in the context of the culture and value systems in which they live and in relation to their goals, expectations, standards, and concerns'. In the Chinese context, the opportunity to fulfil filial responsibilities provides compensation to caregivers by enhancing their spiritual integrity. On the other hand, Patterson et al. (1998) noted that filial discourses suppressing the disclosure of stress and negative feelings about caregiving might have a negative impact on the quality of life for informal caregivers. In any case, according to numerous other scholars, such as Xiao et al. (2014) and Ikels (2004), filial piety is likely to be a very important incentive and motivation for Chinese people to take care of elderly parents.

Decline in Care Practice and Governmental Response

Due to the contextual changes and various forms of care burdens, informal caregivers, especially migrant peasant workers, may encounter more difficulties in sustaining care for their elder parents. Migrant peasant workers' elderly parents are left behind in the rural areas and are in need of care from their children, especially when the parents are not well.

Distance, along with other factors such as access to unpaid leave, financial means, and so on, makes it technically difficult for migrant peasant workers to take care of their parents. Research has shown a decline in care behaviour from migrant peasant workers towards their parents (for example, Ikels, 2004; Koshy, 2013; Nylan, 1996; Poškaitė, 2014; Wang, 2016; Xu, 2012).

In July 2013, the Chinese government published a law enabling parents to sue their children for not visiting regularly, in the name of preserving a part of the essence of Chinese traditional culture: filial piety (which, as previously noted, requires children to care for, respect, and obey their parents; Hatton, 2013). The law is seen as a top-down reaction to the decline of caring behaviours of adult children towards their elderly parents. In response to this decline, both the Chinese government and the general public have more recently shown signs of embracing a social movement to revive Chinese traditional culture and philosophy, with filial piety as a major focus of this movement (Billioud & Thoraval, 2007; Guan, 2005; Song, 2015).

Conclusion

Migrant peasant workers have been recognised as particularly strongly affected by China's neoliberal contextual changes following on from the 1978 economic reforms and are therefore a suitable demographic group on which to focus this exploration. Due to the unique social status of the chosen demographic group, many care burdens, which may or may not be exacerbated by the contextual factors in China, have been identified and are explained. In the next chapter, filial piety is articulated and discussed in relation to my research.

References

Albany, N. Y. (2013, April 22). *China aged care industry & rare earth industry 2012–2015 new market research report* (2013, July 9). Researchmoz. Retrieved from http://www.prweb.com/releases/2013/4/prweb10655868.htm on October 10, 2019.

Aoun, S. M., Bentley, B., Funk, L., Toye, C., Grande, G., & Stajduhar, K. J. (2013). A 10-year literature review of family caregiving for motor neurone disease: Moving from caregiver burden studies to palliative care interventions.

Palliative Medicine, 27(5), 437–446. https://doi.org/10.1177/0269216312455729

Aoun, S. M., Deas, K., Toye, C., Ewing, G., Grande, G., & Stajduhar, K. (2015). Supporting family caregivers to identify their own needs in end-of-life care: Qualitative findings from a stepped wedge cluster trial. *Palliative Medicine, 29*(6), 508–517. https://doi.org/10.1177/0269216314566061

Applebaum, A. J., & Breitbart, W. (2013). Care for the cancer caregiver: A systematic review. *Palliative & Supportive Care, 11*(3), 231–252. https://doi.org/10.1017/S1478951512000594

Babiarz, K. S., Miller, G., Yi, H., Zhang, L., & Rozelle, S. (2010). New evidence on the impact of China's New Rural Cooperative Medical Scheme and its implications for rural primary healthcare: Multivariate difference-in-difference analysis. *British Medical Journal, 341*, c5617. https://doi.org/10.1136/bmj.c5617

Barusch, A. S. (1995). Programming for family care of elderly dependents: Mandates, incentives, and service rationing. *Social Work, 40*(3), 315–322. https://doi.org/10.1093/sw/40.3.315

Billioud, S., & Thoraval, J. (2007). Jiaohua: The Confucian revival in China as an educative project. *China Perspectives, 4*, 4–20. https://journals.openedition.org/Chinaperspectives/

Blot, W. J., Li, J. Y., Taylor, P. R., Guo, W., Dawsey, S., Wang, G. Q., Yang, C. S., Zheng, S. F., Gail, M., Li, G. Y., Yu, Y., Liu, B. Q., Tangrea, J., Sun, Y. H., Liu, F. S., Fraumeni, J. F., Zhang, Y. H., Jr., & Li, B. (1993). Nutrition intervention trials in Linxian, China: Supplementation with specific vitamin/mineral combinations, cancer incidence, and disease-specific mortality in the general population. *Journal of the National Cancer Institute, 85*(18), 1483–1491. https://doi.org/10.1093/jnci/85.18.1483

Blumenthal, D., & Hsiao, W. (2015). Lessons from the East: China's rapidly evolving health care system. *New England Journal of Medicine, 372*(14), 1281–1285. https://doi.org/10.1056/NEJMp1410425

Burns, L. R., & Liu, G. G. (2017). *China's healthcare system and reform*. http://ldi.upenn.edu/sites/default/files/burns-liu-new-China-book.pdf

Cai, Y. (2010). China's below-replacement fertility: Government policy or socioeconomic development? *Population and Development Review, 36*(3), 419–440. https://doi.org/10.1111/j.1728-4457.2010.00341.x

Chan, C. L., Ho, A. H., Leung, P. P., Chochinov, H. M., Neimeyer, R. A., Pang, S. M., & Tse, D. M. (2012). The blessings and the curses of filial piety on dignity at the end-of-life: Lived experience of Hong Kong Chinese adult children caregivers. *Journal of Ethnic and Cultural Diversity in Social Work, 21*(4), 277–296. https://doi.org/10.1080/15313204.2012.729177

Chang, K. S. (1994). Chinese urbanization and development before and after economic reform: A comparative reappraisal. *World Development, 22*(4), 601–613. https://doi.org/10.1016/0305-750X(94)90115-5

Chen, S. (2009). Aging with Chinese characteristics: A public policy perspective. *Ageing International, 34*(3), 172–188. https://doi.org/10.1007/s12126-009-9043-6

Chen, W., Zheng, R., Baade, P. D., Zhang, S., Zeng, H., Bray, F., Jemal, A., Yu, X. Q., & He, J. (2016). Cancer statistics in China, 2015. *A Cancer Journal for Clinicians, 66*(2), 115–132. https://doi.org/10.3322/caac.21338

Chou, R. J. A. (2011). Filial piety by contract? The emergence, implementation, and implications of the "family support agreement" in China. *The Gerontologist, 51*(1), 3–16. https://doi.org/10.1093/geront/gnq059

Cohen, J., & Deliens, L. (2012). *A public health perspective on end-of-life care*. Oxford University Press.

Cohen, S. A., Cook, S., Kelley, L., Sando, T., & Bell, A. E. (2015). Psychosocial factors of caregiver burden in child caregivers: Results from the new national study of caregiving. *Health and Quality of Life Outcomes, 13*(1), 120. https://doi.org/10.1186/s12955-015-0317-2

Cong, Y. (2004). Doctor-family-patient relationship: The Chinese paradigm of informed consent. *The Journal of Medicine and Philosophy, 29*(2), 149–178. https://doi.org/10.1076/jmep.29.2.149.31506

Contro, N., Larson, J., Scofield, S., Sourkes, B., & Cohen, H. (2002). Family perspectives on the quality of pediatric palliative care. *Archives of Pediatrics & Adolescent Medicine, 156*(1), 14–19. https://doi.org/10.3390/children2010131

Corden, A., & Hirst, M. (2011). Partner care at the end-of-life: Identity, language and characteristics. *Ageing & Society, 31*(2), 217–242. https://doi.org/10.1017/S0144686X10000838

Diamond, T. (2009). *Making gray gold: Narratives of nursing home care*. University of Chicago Press.

Disability Support Services. (2018, August 2). *Disability Support Services operational policy*. https://www.health.govt.nz/our-work/disability-services/contracting-and-working-disability-support-services/disability-support-services-operational-policy

Fang, H., Jhing, H., & Lin, C. (2009). Ethical issues in the practice of advance directives, living wills, and self-determination in end-of-life care. *The Journal of Nursing, 56*(1), 17–22. http://xbbjb.nwnu.edu.cn

Feng, W., Cai, Y., & Gu, B. (2013). Population, policy, and politics: How will history judge China's one-child policy? *Population and Development Review, 38*(s1), 115–129. https://www.jstor.org/stable/23655290

Gallagher-Thompson, D., Tzuang, Y. M., Au, A., Brodaty, H., Charlesworth, G., Gupta, R., Lee, S., Losada, S., & Shyu, Y.-I. (2012). International perspectives on nonpharmacological best practices for dementia family caregivers: A review. *Clinical Gerontologist, 35*(4), 316–355. https://doi.org/10.1080/07317115.2012.678190

Gao, Y., Su, B., & Gao, F. (2012). New rural pension system of China: Is it possible? An exploratory study of Feidong County, Anhui Province. *Journal of Cambridge Studies, 7*(3), 122–132. https://doi.org/10.17863/CAM.1446

Gong, P., Liang, S., Carlton, E. J., Jiang, Q., Wu, J. Y., Wang, L., & Remais, J. V. (2012). Urbanisation and health in China. *The Lancet, 379*(9818), 843–852. https://doi.org/10.1016/S0140-6736(11)61878-3

Gruijters, R. J. (2017). Family care-giving and living arrangements of functionally impaired elders in rural China. *Ageing and Society, 37*(3), 633–647. https://doi.org/10.1017/S0144686X15001397

Guan, Y. (2005). Legal protection for traditional knowledge and traditional culture expressions "传统知识及传统文化表达的法律保护问题". *Normal University of Guizhou University Press (Social Science), 2*(3), 14–26. http://www.gznu.edu.cn

Hancock, K., Clayton, J. M., Parker, S. M., Walder, S., Butow, P. N., Carrick, S., Currow, D., Ghersi, P., Hagerty, R., & Tattersall, M. H. N. (2007). Truth-telling in discussing prognosis in advanced life-limiting illnesses: A systematic review. *Palliative Medicine, 21*(6), 507–517. http://journals.sagepub.com/home/pmj

Hatton, C. (2013, August 8). New China law says children "must visit parents". *BBC News*. http://www.bbc.com/news/world-asia-China-23124345

He, L., & van Heugten, K. (2020). Chinese migrant workers' care experiences: A model of the mediating roles of filial piety. *Qualitative Health Research, 30*(11), 1–13. https://doi.org/10.1177/1049732320925420

Hesketh, T., Lu, L., & Xing, Z. W. (2005). The effect of China's one-child family policy after 25 years. *The New England Journal of Medicine, 353*(11), 1171–1176. https://doi.org/10.1056/NEJMhpr051833

Hooyman, N. R., & Kiyak, H. A. (2008). Opportunities and challenges of informal caregiving. In N. R. Hooyman & H. A. Kiyak (Eds.), *Social gerontology: A multidisciplinary perspective* (pp. 385–428). Allyn & Bacon.

Hu, B., Li, B., Wang, J., & Shi, C. (2020). Home and community care for older people in urban China: Receipt of services and sources of payment. *Health & Social Care in the Community, 28*(1), 225–235. https://doi.org/10.1111/hsc.12856

Huang, Y. (2018). Changing intergenerational contracts: Gender, cohorts and elder care in central rural China, 2005–2013. *Asian Population Studies, 14*(1), 5–21. https://doi.org/10.1080/17441730.2017.1341090

Ikels, C. (2004). *Filial piety: Practice and discourse in contemporary East Asia*. Stanford University Press.

Jackson, S., & Liu, J. (2017). The social context of ageing and intergenerational relationships in Chinese families. *The Journal of Chinese Sociology, 4*(1), 1–5. https://doi.org/10.1186/s40711-016-0050-1

Jiang, Y., Liu, C., Li, J. Y., Huang, M. J., Yao, W. X., Zhang, R., Yao, B., Du, X. B., Chen, J., Xie, K., Zhao, X., & Wei, Y. Q. (2007). Different attitudes of Chinese patients and their families towards truth telling of different stages of cancer. *Psycho-Oncology, 16*(10), 928–936. https://doi.org/10.1002/pon.1156

Joseph, A. E., & Phillips, D. R. (1999). Ageing in rural China: Impacts of increasing diversity in family and community resources. *Journal of Cross-Cultural Gerontology, 14*(2), 153–168. https://doi.org/10.1023/A:1006658706496

Jung, J., & Liu Streeter, J. (2015). Does health insurance decrease health expenditure risk in developing countries? The case of China. *Southern Economic Journal, 82*(2), 361–384. https://doi.org/10.1002/soej.12101

Kendall, S. (2006). Being asked not to tell: Nurses' experiences of caring for cancer patients not told their diagnosis. *Journal of Clinical Nursing, 15*(9), 1149–1157. https://doi.org/10.1111/j.1365-2702.2006.01460.x

Kortes-Miller, K. (2015). OA6 talking about death won't kill you; introducing die-alogues. *British Medical Journal Supportive & Palliative Care, 5*(Suppl. 1), A2. https://spcare.bmj.com/content/5/Suppl_1/A2.3.short

Koshy, S. (2013). Neoliberal family matters. *American Literary History, 25*(2), 344–380. https://doi.org/10.1093/alh/ajt006

Li, M., Mao, W., Chi, I., & Lou, V. W. Q. (2019). Geographical proximity and depressive symptoms among adult child caregivers: Social support as a moderator. *Aging & Mental Health, 23*(2), 205–213. https://doi.org/10.1080/13607863.2017.1399349

Li, Y., Wu, Q., Xu, L., Legge, D., Hao, Y., Gao, L., Ning, N., & Wan, G. (2012). Factors affecting catastrophic health expenditure and impoverishment from medical expenses in China: Policy implications of universal health insurance. *Bulletin of the World Health Organization, 90*(9), 664–671.

Lin, X. (2013). *Gender, modernity and male migrant workers in China: Becoming a "modern" man*. Routledge.

Lin, Y., Hu, C., Xu, Y., Zhao, J., & Li, Q. (2020). The mutual impact and moderating factors of quality of life between advanced cancer patients and their family caregivers. *Supportive Care in Cancer, 28*, 5251–5262. https://doi.org/10.1007/s00520-020-05351-x

Liu, J., Cheng, Y., Lau, J. F. L., Anise, W. M. S., Tse, V. S., & Zhou, S. L. (2015). The majority of the migrant factory workers of the light industry in

Shenzhen, China may be physically inactive. *PLoS ONE, 10*(8), e0131734. https://doi.org/10.1371/journal.pone.0131734

Liu, L. (2004). Chuanshan theory's evolution, difficulty, and future 百年船山学的变迁、困境与出路. *Nantong Normal University Publisher: Social Science Edition* 南通师范学院学报:哲学社会科学版, *20*(1), 149–153. https://www.21ks.net/shkx/shkx_15628.html

Liu, T., & Sun, L. (2016). Pension reform in China. *Journal of Aging & Social Policy, 28*(1), 15–28. https://doi.org/10.1080/08959420.2016.1111725

Liu, Z.-W., Yu, Y., Fang, L., Hu, M., Zhou, L., & Xiao, S.-Y. (2019). Willingness to receive institutional and community-based eldercare among the rural elderly in China. *PLoS ONE, 14*(11), e0225314. https://doi.org/10.1371/journal.pone.0225314

Lu, L., Pan, B., Sun, W., Cheng, L., Chi, T., Chi, T. S., & Wang, L. (2010). Quality of life and related factors among cancer caregivers in China. *Psychiatry and Clinical Neurosciences, 64*(5), 505–513. https://doi.org/10.1111/j.1440-1819.2010.02131.x

Ma, H. (2015). A pragmatic study of the influence of average income on consumption in rural China 农村人均收入对消费影响的实证研究——基于中国农村居民人均收入与消费的分析. *Tianjing Business Vocational College Publication* 天津商务职业学院学报, *3*(5), 5–10. http://xb.tcc1955.edu.cn/

Mao, W. Y. (2010). Well-being of caregivers to older adults in China. *USC US-China Institute, 23*(5), 33–37. https://China.usc.edu/

Meier, D. (2012). *Palliative care: Deploying mindfulness to transform the care of serious illness.* Paper presented at the Buddhist Contemplative Care Symposium, New York Zen Center for Contemplative Care and the Garrison Institute, New York, NY.

Meng, A. (2013). Informal home care and labor-force participation of household members. *Empirical Economics, 44*(2), 959–979. https://doi.org/10.1007/s00181-011-0537-1

Ngai, P., & Huilin, L. (2010). Unfinished proletarianization: Self, anger, and class action among the second generation of peasant-workers in present-day China. *Modern China, 36*(5), 493–519. http://journals.sagepub.com/home/mcx

Nylan, M. (1996). Confucian piety and individualism in Han China. *Journal of the American Oriental Society, 116*(1), 1–27. https://doi.org/10.2307/606369

OECD. (2012). Pensions at a glance Asia/Pacific 2011. *OECD iLibrary*. https://doi.org/10.1787/9789264107007-en

Palm, E. (2013). Who cares? Moral obligations in formal and informal care provision in the light of ICT-based home care. *Health Care Analysis, 21*(2), 171–188. https://link.springer.com/journal/10728

Pan, W., & Feng, X. (2007). Family caregivers' real life experiences of terminal cancer 晚期癌症患者亲属照顾者的真实生活体验. *China Modern Nursing, 1*(2), 20–30. 中华现代护理学杂志.

Papastavrou, E., Charalambous, A., & Tsangari, H. (2009). Exploring the other side of cancer care: The informal caregiver. *European Journal of Oncology Nursing, 13*(2), 128–136. http://www.medsci.cn/sci/journal.do?id=9c7510161

Patterson, T. L., Semple, S., Shaw, W., Yu, E., He, Y., Zhang, M., Wu, W., & Grant, I. (1998). The cultural context of caregiving: A comparison of Alzheimer's caregivers in Shanghai, China and San Diego, California. *Psychological Medicine, 28*(5), 1071–1084. http://www.letpub.com.cn

Phillips, J. E., Ajrouch, K. J., & Hillcoat-Nallétamby, S. (2010). *Key concepts in social gerontology*. Sage.

Pizzo, P., Walker, D., & Bomba, P. (2015). *Dying in America: Improving quality and honoring individual preferences near the end-of-life*. Institute of Medicine.

Poškaitė, L. (2014). Filial piety (xiao 孝) for the contemporary and global world. *Asian Studies, 2*(1), 99–114. https://doi.org/10.4312/as.2014.2.1.99-114

PRWeb. (2013, April 22). *China aged care industry & rare earth industry 2012–2015 new market research report available at Researchmoz*. http://www.prweb.com/releases/2013/4/prweb10655868.htm

Rehman, L., Reading, C., & Unruh, A. (2009). "You grow from it … you get more spiritual": An exploration of spirituality, health, and leisure for unpaid caregivers. *Leisure/Loisir, 33*(1), 367–388. https://doi.org/10.1080/14927713.2009.9651443

Rofel, L. (2007). *Desiring China: Experiments in neoliberalism, sexuality, and public culture*. Duke University Press.

Salditt, F., Whiteford, P., & Adema, W. (2007). Pension reform in China. *International Social Security Review, 61*(3), 47–71. https://doi.org/10.1111/j.1468-246X.2008.00316.x

Seo, Y. J., & Park, H. (2019). Factors influencing caregiver burden in families of hospitalised patients with lung cancer. *Journal of Clinical Nursing, 28*(9–10), 1979–1989. https://doi.org/10.1111/jocn.14812

Shi, C., & Hu, B. (2020). Preferences for formal social care in rural and urban China: Evidence from a national survey. *Journal of Gerontological Social Work, 63*(1–2), 19–40. https://doi.org/10.1080/01634372.2019.1709246

Social Security Official Website. (2017). *2017 New Rural Cooperative Health Scheme reimbursement rate and guidelines*. http://www.chashebao.com/yiliaobaoxian/17737.html

Song, Z. (2015). From "accordingly" to "expanding": A discussion of Feng Youlan's new thoughts on Confucianism 从"照着讲"到"接着讲"——论冯友兰讲儒学的新思路. *Social Science Frontline* (2), 9–16.

Tang, S., Ehiri, J., & Long, Q. (2013). China's biggest, most neglected health challenge: Non-communicable diseases. *Infectious Diseases of Poverty, 2*(1), 7–7. https://doi.org/10.1186/2049-9957-2-7

Terry, Y. S. L., Elsie, C. W. Y., Andy, H. Y. H., Michelle, H. Y. S., Gloria, H. Y. W., Mandy, M. Y. L., & Wang, J. (2016). Measuring filial piety in the 21st century. *Journal of Applied Gerontology, 35*(11), 1235–1247. https://doi.org/10.1177/0733464815570664

Tse, C., Chong, A., & Fok, S. (2003). Breaking bad news: A Chinese perspective. *Palliative Medicine, 17*(4), 339–343. https://doi.org/10.1191/0269216303pm751oa

Ugalde, A., Krishnasamy, M., & Schofield, P. (2012). Role recognition and changes to self-identity in family caregivers of people with advanced cancer: A qualitative study. *Supportive Care in Cancer, 20*(6), 1175–1181. https://doi.org/10.1007/s00520-011-1194-9

Wang, F. L. (2016). Institutions and institutional change in China: Premodernity and modernization. *American Political Science Review, 94*(2), 498–499. https://doi.org/10.2307/2586081

Wang, F., Peng, X., & Gu, B. (2011). *Globalization and low birth rate: The choice of China* [全球化与低生育率:中国的选择] (Dissertation). Fudan University, Shanghai.

Wang, L., Kong, L., Wu, F., Bai, Y., & Burton, R. (2005). Preventing chronic diseases in China. *The Lancet, 366*(9499), 1821–1824. https://doi.org/10.1016/S0140-6736(05)67344-8

Wang, Y., Shi, Z., Li, Y., & Du, Q. (2014). Analysis of nurse absence in comprehensive hospital level 3A 三级甲等综合医院护士缺岗原因分析. *Nursing Magazine* 护理学杂志, *29*(7), 14–16. http://www.hlxzz.com.cn/ch/index.aspx

Williamson, J. B., Fang, L., & Calvo, E. (2017). Rural pension reform in China: A critical analysis. *Journal of Aging Studies, 41*, 67–74. https://doi.org/10.1016/j.jaging.2017.04.003

Williamson, J. B., Price, M., & Shen, C. (2012). Pension policy in China, Singapore, and South Korea: An assessment of the potential value of the notional defined contribution model. *Journal of Aging Studies, 26*(1), 79–89. https://doi.org/10.1016/j.jaging.2011.08.002

Wong, K., Fu, D., Li, C. Y., & Song, H. X. (2007). Rural migrant workers in urban China: Living a marginalised life. *International Journal of Social Welfare, 16*(1), 32–40. https://doi.org/10.1111/j.1468-2397.2007.00475.x

World Health Organization. (2015). *People's Republic of China health system review*. Manila, Philippines: WHO Regional Office for the Western Pacific. https://www.who.int/iris/handle/10665/208229

World Health Organisation. (n.d.-a). *Cancer: WHO definition of palliative care*. Geneva, Switzerland. http://www.who.int/cancer/palliative/definition/en/

World Health Organisation. (n.d.-b). *WHOQOL: Measuring quality of life*. Geneva, Switzerland: Author. Retrieved from http://www.who.int/healthinfo/survey/whoqol-qualityoflife/en/

Wu, B., Mao, Z., & Xu, Q. (2008). Institutional care for elders in rural China. *Journal of Aging & Social Policy, 20*(2), 218–239. https://doi.org/10.1080/08959420801977632

Xiao, L. D., Wang, J., He, G.-P., De Bellis, A., Verbeeck, J., & Kyriazopoulos, H. (2014). Family caregiver challenges in dementia care in Australia and China: A critical perspective. *BMC Geriatrics, 14*(1), 6–6. https://doi.org/10.1186/1471-2318-14-6

Xing, H. (2015). Seven questions about the catastrophic health insurance 七问"大病医保". *Rural, Agriculture, Peasants* 农村·农业·农民, *1*(8), 14–15.

Xu, J. (2012). Filial piety and intergenerational communication in China: A nationwide study. *Journal of International Communication, 18*(1), 33–48. https://doi.org/10.1080/13216597.2012.662466

Xu, Y., Wu, Y., Zhang, Y., Ma, R., & Li, X. (2016). Caregiver human resource national investigation 全国医院护士人力资源现状的调查. *China Caregiving Magazine* 中华护理杂志, *51*(7), 819–822. http://zh.zhhlzzs.com/CN/0254-1769/home.shtml

Xu, Z. Y., Blot, W. J., Xiao, H.-P., Wu, A., Feng, Y. P., Stone, B. J., Sun, J., Ershow, A. G., Henderson, B. E., & Fraumeni, J. F. (1989). Smoking, air pollution, and the high rates of lung cancer in Shenyang, China. *JNCI: Journal of the National Cancer Institute, 81*(23), 1800–1806. https://academic.oup.com/jnci

Ye, J. Z., Wang, C. Y., Wu, H. F., He, C. Z., & Liu, J. (2013). Internal migration and left-behind populations in China. *The Journal of Peasant Studies, 40*(6), 1119–1146. https://doi.org/10.1080/03066150.2013.861421

Yi, Z., & George, L. K. (2010). Population ageing and old-age insurance in China. In D. Dannefer & C. Phillipson (Eds.), *The SAGE handbook of social gerontology* (pp. 420–429). Sage. https://doi.org/10.4135/9781446200933.n32

Yick, A. G., & Gupta, R. (2002). Chinese cultural dimensions of death, dying, and bereavement: Focus group findings. *Journal of Cultural Diversity, 9*(2), 32–42. http://tuckerpub.com/jcd.htm

Zeng, Y., Land, K. C., Gu, D., & Wang, Z. (2013). *Household and living arrangement projections: The extended cohort-component method and applications to the US and China*. Springer.

Zhang, H. (2019). Sending parents to nursing homes is unfilial? An exploratory study on institutional elder care in China. *International Social Work, 62*(1), 351–362. https://doi.org/10.1177/0020872817725137

Zhang, K. H., & Shunfeng, S. (2003). Rural–urban migration and urbanization in China: Evidence from time-series and cross-section analyses. *China Economic Review, 14*(4), 386–400. https://doi.org/10.1016/j.chieco.2003.09.018

Zhang, L. Y., Cheng, X. M., Tolhurst, R., Tang, S. L., & Liu, X. Y. (2010). How effectively can the new cooperative medical scheme reduce catastrophic health expenditure for the poor and non-poor in rural China? *Tropical Medicine & International Health, 15*(4), 468–475. https://doi.org/10.1111/j.1365-3156.2010.02469.x

Zhang, N. J., Guo, M., & Zheng, X. Y. (2012). China: Awakening giant developing solutions to population aging. *The Gerontologist, 52*(5), 589–596. https://doi.org/10.1093/geront/gns105

Zhu, L. (2001). Collective discrimination and bias: The conflicting interaction between migrant peasant workers and urban residents 群体性偏见与歧视--农民工与市民的磨擦性互动. *Jianghai Academic Periodical* 江海学刊 (6), 48–53.

Zimmer, Z. (2016). *Global ageing in the twenty-first century: Challenges, opportunities and implications*. Routledge.

CHAPTER 2

A Historical Trajectory of Filial Piety

Introduction

As was clear during my fieldwork, filial piety is an extremely important discourse influencing migrant peasant workers' care practices and experiences. Filial piety in China is a philosophical, social, economic, cultural, traditional, moral, and political guideline, discourse, knowledge system, and priority. It was originally centred in Chinese familial relationships and later extended to the relationship between the state and its people. As a profound cultural norm, filial piety was identified as needing to be at the core of the research design before fieldwork commenced, although I had not imagined it would be as central to the participants' subjective construction of their care experiences as the interviews eventually revealed it to be.

Filial piety has evolved continuously since it was elevated by Confucius over 2,000 years ago as a philosophical, theoretical, and ethical concept and as a core value. The concept has developed over several stages that somewhat followed the dynastic periods. The Confucian and neo-Confucian periods were most crucial to this development and are therefore explained in more detail in this chapter. During the New Culture Movement (1910s–1920s) and Cultural Revolution (1966–1976), filial piety and Confucianism were heavily criticised and western modernisation was established as the primary goal for the state (although in between these reform periods it quickly regained its strength and received renewed

L. He, *Care Work, Migrant Peasant Families and Discourse of Filial Piety in China*, https://doi.org/10.1007/978-981-16-1880-2_2

scholarly attention). Since China's economic reform in 1978, there has been a tendency to attribute diminishing filial practices to neoliberalism (Ikels, 2004; Koshy, 2013; Rofel, 2007; Trnka & Trundle, 2014). This chapter partially adopts a Foucauldian genealogical way of understanding filial piety by delving into its historical trajectory, of which I will focus a few important eras.

Eastern Zhou Dynasty, Spring and Autumn Period and Warring States Period, and the Contention of a Hundred Schools of Thought (770–221 BCE)

The time of the Eastern Zhou dynasty included the Spring and Autumn period followed by the Warring States period. Chinese society was facing socio-economic turmoil as the old social order collapsed with a new order not yet established (Liu, 2013). A number of great philosophers and thinkers emerged who engaged in tackling unsettling social issues through their theories and ideals. A great range of ideas flourished throughout that period, later called the Contention of a Hundred Schools of Thought. Each of these great thinkers and ideologists endeavoured to make the particular vassal state in which they lived and worked prosperous and strong (Liu, 2013). Although these thinkers had different takes on many moral and ethical issues, filial piety was positively recognised by almost all of them even while reflecting different focuses and interpretations. Here I briefly consider Confucianism and two other schools as examples of how different theorists at that time constructed filial piety.

Confucianism

Eldercare and filial behaviours emerged long before the Eastern Zhou dynasty (Luo, 2013). After the teachings of the first and most influential Confucianist, Confucius (551–479 BCE), filial behaviours and 'raw' affection between parents and children were elevated to become filial piety, which became a behavioural regulation, a moral guideline, an everyday life principle, a governing ideology, and a fundamental philosophy (Ikels, 2004; Poškaitė, 2014; Xu, 2012).

One focus of the teaching of Confucius was the art of governance, the aim of which was the maintenance of a proper social order (Ames &

Rosemont, 2010; Chen, 2002). On the other hand, Confucius accentuated the notions of proper ways of behaviour and of the need to pursue self-cultivation to become a worthy and 'complete' human being (Chen, 2002). For Confucius, morality and ethics existed and were evidenced in the conduct of appropriate social relations and self-cultivation (J. Li, 2003a). Morality was the essence of governance of both society and the self (J. Li, 2003a). As the first private educator, Confucius taught many who went on to serve for different governments (Feng, 1995). Later on, from the Han dynasty (202 BCE–220 CE) until the last dynasty, the Qing (1644–1911), Confucianism represented and became an ideological governing tool for the unity of the Chinese empire ("Neo-Confucianism", 2016). Confucianism itself evolved throughout history (Goldin, 2011). According to St. André (2018), filial piety has consistently been the foundation of all virtues in Confucian philosophy; filiality has been consistently regarded as an irrefutable component of human morality (Ikels, 2004).

Taoism

The founder of philosophical Taoism, Laozi (ca. 604–ca. 531 BCE), argued that relinquishing righteousness and benevolence and returning to nature would ensure that filiality and kind-heartedness would return (Luo, 2013). He proposed a state of complete freedom of thinking, away from the constraints of social morality (Zhang, 2009). However, Laozi never negatively criticised the support and nourishing of one's elders (Luo, 2013). According to Zhang (2009), Taoism might appear to have involved a period of time when the Confucian notion of filial piety was rejected, as it rejected the inequality of filial power between parents and children. However, Taoism embraced the provision of care and the emotional bond between parents and children (Luo, 2013). Zhang (2009) wrote about the similarity between Confucian and Taoist views of filial piety in terms of filial care and intergenerational bonds, and explained that the difference lay in the Taoist disagreement with the hierarchical principle of 'obedience', whereby children needed to obey and respect their parents unquestioningly.

From the Song to the Qing Dynasty (960–1912 CE)

Filial piety was an important foundation stone for economic and social improvements during the dynasties that preceded the Song dynasty (Luo,

2013). As Li and Nie (2012) stated, it solved the problem of low social trust before the Han dynasty. Through filial piety, society formed a system of trust and stability, on the basis of which economic activities could take place peacefully. As a means to maintaining feudal rule and economic productivity, filial piety played its role brilliantly from the Han dynasty to the Tang dynasty (618–907 CE; Li & Nie, 2012). However, the massive patriarchal family system—which determined the governance of large tracts of land, monopolised the social economy, and was involved in the distribution of political privilege during those times—was significantly altered by various uprisings and wars at the end of the Tang dynasty (Luo & Wang, 2013). From the Song dynasty (960–1279) to the Qing dynasty (1616–1912), small landlords and free peasants increasingly emerged. At the same time, many handicraft workshops and markets blossomed in the cities (Luo & Wang, 2013). The social structure for filial piety built up over a thousand years from the Han dynasty to the Tang dynasty was destroyed. Thus, a new school of thought (neo-Confucianism) emerged, and the discourse of filial piety changed accordingly (Luo, 2013).

Neo-Confucianism

Neo-Confucianism emerged during the Tang dynasty and flourished during the Song dynasty (Luo, 2013). Neo-Confucianism was founded in response to the stagnation of traditional Confucianism and concerns over the dominance of the foreign religion of Buddhism, which had been introduced from India (Feng, 1995). Politically, reforms were also considered to be required to tackle socio-economic changes resulting from, for example, constant wars and the dissolving of large-scale patriarchal family systems. Neo-Confucianism responded to these challenges by reinterpreting ancient Confucian traditions (Foster, 2014). It tried to introduce certain basic elements of Buddhist spirituality and Taoist cosmology into Confucianism. Confucianism, which accentuated governmentality through building a social morality and through study, was regarded as a suitable complement to Buddhism's spirituality and more profound metaphysical ideas about the universe (Feng, 1995). For example, the approach to achieving self-cultivation through Buddhist meditation was much more appealing than the Confucian approach, which required schooling and self-discipline. Confucian ethics and philosophy were revised to incorporate metaphysical and cosmological ideas from Buddhism and Taoism (Foster, 2014). Neo-Confucianism did not simply borrow the spiritual expectations and ascetical philosophy from Buddhism but reinterpreted ancient Confucianism to meet new philosophical and spiritual challenges (Feng, 1995). The ascetical doctrine was amended to incorporate pathways for self-cultivation and eventual self-transformation, culminating in the achievement of *agehood*.

Wrongdoing/Negative Effects of Neo-Confucianism and Filial Piety

In the neo-Confucian discourse, everyone had to follow moral and ethical guidelines according to *li* (principle), which dictates a way of conduct for every scenario (Luo, 2013). Such assertions decreed *sangang wuchang* (三纲五常)—three cardinal guides and five constant virtues—as specific moral principles to be obeyed. The three cardinal guides stipulated that the ruler guides the subject, the father guides the son, and the husband guides the wife. The five constant virtues were righteousness, propriety, sincerity, knowledge, and benevolence (You, 2006). These moral principles essentialised and magnified the 'obedience'-focused aspect of filial piety. Through *sangang wuchang*, people's natural desire and creativity were smothered (Feng, 1995; You, 2006). Neo-Confucianists were encouraged to promote these discursive principles in their education programmes (You, 2006; Zhu, 1999).

The thriving of neo-Confucianism and the government's strong emphasis on filial piety led to numerous simplistic approaches to filial practices (Luo & Wang, 2013). The government engaged in extensive propaganda to promote filial piety through a focus on moral examples (Tang & Li, 2001). While some of the exemplary stories contained community-enhancing morals, others encouraged extremism that overstepped common behavioural boundaries. There are, for example, reports of purportedly historical events in which children cut their own flesh to feed their ill parents as a form of medical treatment or took revenge on a parent's murderer by killing them in turn. For the latter action, the children apparently not only escaped trial but also received positive recognition from the government, all in the name of filial piety. Of course, as Tang and Li (2001) suggested, rather than reflecting real events these stories may have been told as parables to highlight exemplary morality.

The promotion of these principles led to an extreme imbalance of power relations between generations (Tang & Li, 2001). Within neo-Confucian discourse parents could exercise absolute power over their children because children had to show them unquestioning obedience.

The killing of one's own children, even, was not considered a crime in many areas during the Qing dynasty (Tang & Li, 2001). According to Ikels (2004) and You (2006), through the discursive practice of neo-Confucian filial piety, the idea that the emperor is the 'father of all' was imposed to enforce people complying with filial obligations towards the emperor as they would towards their own parents; thus, loyalty towards the emperor became highly magnified (Ikels, 2004; Luo, 2013). Filial discourse constructed a hierarchical system from the central government to the local level through the promotion of filial piety and the punishment of unfilial and disobedient behaviours (Luo, 2013).

Chapter 4 considers how neo-Confucian filial discourse resembled a western modern space where (scientific) disciplinary power is practised and exercised, as Foucault described in his book *The Archaeology of Knowledge* (Foucault, 1970). This kind of disciplinary power was exercised everywhere through neo-Confucian filial discourse, and it became stricter and more controlling over time.

From the End of the Qing Dynasty (Late Nineteenth Century) to the Cultural Revolution (1966–1976)

From the end of the Qing dynasty, China's revolutionary task was to achieve national independence from western invasion and influence (Luk, 1989). A number of scholars and young intellectuals were determined to learn from the west while at the same time defending China against western invasion and colonisation. The traditional Chinese neo-Confucian ethics of *sangang wuchang* were heavily criticised (Luk, 1989). At the same time, there were also scholars who endeavoured to confront and respond to mainstream criticism and reconstruct filial piety in such a way as to adapt to a western ideal of modernity (X. Li, 2003; Z. Zhang, 2017).

New Culture Movement (1910s–1920s) and New Confucianism (from the Early Twentieth Century)

The May Fourth Movement (1919) saw an uprising led by Chinese students in a comprehensive move against neo-Confucian filial piety, which was labelled as feudal (Li, 2014). The movement embraced democracy and sought to abandon Confucianism as the mainstream ideology

(X. Li, 2003b, 2014). The New Culture Movement also emerged during this time (1910s–1920s) but was mainly led by scholars rather than students (X. Li, 2003b). One of the most influential representatives, Chen Duxiu (1887–1942), who became the founder and main early leader of the Chinese Communist Party, established the magazine *New Youth*, which fiercely criticised and repelled Confucianism and traditional filial culture. The New Culture Movement ended the dominant position of Confucianism in mainstream academia in China for many years (X. Li, 2003b).

As the core value of Confucianism, filial piety was significantly negatively impacted for the first time in thousands of years (Luo, 2013). According to Luo (2013), Chen Duxiu once said that the essence of *sangang wuchang* was to emphasise obligation over rights: children only needed to know what they should do, as opposed to what they wanted to do. Chen Duxiu asserted that this ethical ideology was based on a patriarchal clan system and needed to be overturned because it hindered social development and socialist productivity (Luo, 2013). For Chen Duxiu, Confucianism, especially neo-Confucian filial piety, was the culprit responsible for China being defeated and largely colonised by the west (Luo, 2013). He devoted his whole life to promote individualist freedom over duty to the family and to reject Confucian familialism. Hu Shi (1891–1962), another influential scholar from the New Culture Movement, proposed that a son should not listen to everything his parents say but rather should be a person who stands up for himself. Hu Shi believed that a child should only ask for his parents' permission if his parents are virtuous enough to be asked. Hu Shi's idea emphasised an equal power balance between parents and children. The discourse of neo-Confucian intergenerational relationships was thus dismantled.

In promoting these new ideas, Hu Shi introduced a new discourse, one which fiercely rejected filial piety and embraced western individualist freedom. During the New Culture Movement, three aspects of filial piety were targeted for criticism, as outlined by Luo (2013). Firstly, filial piety formed the philosophical and conceptual basis for the outdated forms of governance of a ruling empire through which Chinese people were suppressed and exploited. Secondly, filial piety was seen as preventing children from developing and pursuing their own life goals. Lastly, simple-minded and blind filial practices were strongly rejected, including examples previously promoted as 'ideal', such as feeding ill parents one's own flesh to achieve a cure, doing nothing but crying over one's father's tomb for years, and so on.

According to Luo (2013), however, the criticism of filial piety was ultimately limited. During and after the New Culture Movement, influential scholars such as Kang Youwei (1858–1927) and Chen Huanzhang (1880–1933) called for respect for Confucianism and filial order. These scholars, especially Kang Youwei, were arguably the founders of New Confucianism, which aims to establish a position for Confucianism in modern China (X. Zhang, 2017). The main leader of the Xinhai Revolution and also the founder of the Republic of China (1912–1949), Sun Yat-sen (1866–1925), also agreed that the Chinese people had been attentive and loyal to family values and that this led to a functional and meaningful system starting from close kin and moving to the patriarchal clan and then the state, each following the next in an orderly way (Luo, 2013). However, his compassionate sentiment, as well as that of other revolutionaries, towards Kang and Chen's revitalising of Confucian culture and ideology did not last long (X. Zhang, 2017). Criticism of these virtues continued to build during the New Culture Movement.

New Confucianism

Filial piety was reconstructed to some extent with the emergence of New Confucianism, which stretched from the early twentieth century to the period after China's economic reform. It involved a number of scholars devoted to reconnecting neo-Confucianism with modernity by preserving its cultural essence and discarding its feudal ethics. However, New Confucianists of the early twentieth century could not save filial piety from being cast out of mainstream ideology. Democracy, freedom, and anti-imperialism informed the key discourses of the time. According to X. Zhang (2017), most New Confucianists had to admit that western ideologies and philosophies had overwhelmed Chinese ones and reconstructed Confucianism in the context of Chinese society at that time. Therefore, it was almost inevitable that the Chinese philosophers and social scientists in their mission failed to dissuade the heavy criticism of Confucianism in mainstream society (X. Zhang, 2017).

From the People's Republic of China to Economic Reform in 1978

After the People's Republic of China was founded in 1949, criticism of traditional filial piety reached its peak (Luo, 2013). In my research, I chose the Great Leap Forward (GLF) and Cultural Revolution (CR) as representatives of the period after the People's Republic of China's founding up to a few years after the start of economic reform in 1978. This period symbolises hardship, lack of material resources, and bitterness (*xinku* 辛苦) (Ge, 2016). My participants referred to this period as 'those years'. Since the economic reform, and especially since the end of the 1980s, citizens have been discouraged from focusing too deeply on the GLF and CR (Kraus, 2012; Rosen, 2007). This period is almost considered as taboo in the Foucauldian sense of the concept of taboo, which will be discussed in Chapter 4.

The Great Leap Forward (1958–1962) and the Cultural Revolution (1966–1976)

According to R. Li (2004) and Xi and Jin (2006), both the GLF and the CR were extremely complicated social and political events that cannot be comprehensively explained in a linear and summarised exposition. Nonetheless, to aid general understanding, I provide here a basic introduction to these two events as they are fundamental to the period between the foundation of the People's Republic of China and the initiation of economic reform in 1978.

According to Bachman (2006, p. 2), the GLF was 'a two-year attempt, from early 1958 to the end of 1959, to implement a communist utopia in China... [that] was energized by the belief that through one titanic effort everything could be done at once'. The phrase 'Great Leap Forward' has a number of meanings. Firstly, it can refer to a specific period of time which according to Bachman (2006) be considered to have started as early as 1955, when the Eighth National Congress instigated accelerated economic development. For my research, I chose Peng's (1987) definition of 1958–1962, a period that also included the Great Chinese Famine (1959–1961). The term can also be understood to refer to a strategy of resource allocation and economic development aimed at higher productivity, increasing gross domestic product, higher investment, decentralised production, industrial agriculture, and self-reliance (Bachman, 2006).

MacFarquhar and Mao (1989) proposed that 'GLF' could refer to a state of mind that the state adopted for reaching a utopian goal of building a communist society. These scholars all pointed to the GLF as having led to the famine of 1959–1961, which resulted in a death toll of millions (Bachman, 2006; MacFarquhar & Mao, 1989; Peng, 1987).

The [Great Proletarian] Cultural Revolution (1966–1976) was led by the Chinese Communist Party (Wu, 2013). Its goal was to cleanse and rectify the Chinese bureaucratic system, which it viewed as corrupt. However, the project spun out of control, and a huge proportion of Chinese people ended up entangled in factional fights (Wu, 2013). Kraus (2012, p. 20) described it as follows:

> It was proletarian more in aspiration than in reality, given that four-fifths of Chinese were peasants. It was cultural, in that its most consistent targets were the arts and popular beliefs. It was not in itself a great revolution; it made a lot of noise but only shook up the state—it did not overturn it. Like most revolutions, it overstayed its welcome. It is tempting to regard this raucous decade as the last and perhaps final push in a century-long trajectory of Chinese revolution, after which China got down to the serious business of building a modern nation.

According to Wu (2012), for the generation that experienced the CR, images of madness were burned in their memories. Time may have helped by hiding those images behind more recent experiences, but any reminder can bring these memories back up and cause renewed pain (Wu, 2012).

As claimed by Manning and Wemheuer (2011), although the GLF and the CR need to be seen as separate, they have often been considered together in terms of the hardships and lasting scars they wrought upon Chinese people of that generation. They report that the famine prompted by the GLF took between 15 and 43 million lives, and that after 1962, malnutrition continued to be a major issue, especially among rural Chinese, until the mid-1980s (Manning & Wemheuer, 2011).

During 'those years', the Chinese government led a concerted criticism of Confucianism, and this included filial piety (Yan, 1999). The dominant political discourse determined that anything that symbolised backwardness, that was seen as old-fashioned or non-progressive, should be destroyed (Ge, 2016). Of course, what was more old-fashioned than a social and familial value that had been passed down for thousands of years? Confucian ideals, and in particular filial piety, were thus denied and dismantled (Wang, 2014). Some children became alienated from their parents; for example, sons would publicly defy their fathers for their 'old' ways (Wang, 2014).

As mentioned above, after neo-Confucianism became the mainstream ideology, filial piety had predominantly included a focus on obedience and the provision of care for elders. Mufson (1996) disagreed with the notion that such provision of care was not discouraged by the government during the GLF and CR, clarifying that obedience towards parents, but not obedience towards the government, was discouraged during the GLF and CR. Ji (2004) similarly claimed that the government demanded everyone's obedience to the state and to the communist ideal. Some scholars, such as Ling (1994), who professed that the Chinese government during those years acted as a parental state, similar to a parental figure in Confucian conceptualisations of filial piety. Ling (1994) asserted that the state–society relationship paralleled a filial parent–child relationship, reflecting Confucian filial relationships that favour the parent (state). However, other scholars (e.g., Wang, 2010, 2014) thought Confucian filial piety and other aspects of traditional culture became greatly diminished during the GLF and CR. In any case, most scholars agree that the practice of filial piety at a family and intergenerational level was eroded.

Autonomous Individual Propaganda and the Modernisation Project

During the GLF and CR, the Chinese government also initiated propaganda sympathetic with criticism of Confucianism and filial piety. According to McDaniel and Zimmer (2013), since the foundation of People's Republic of China, the Chinese government has had a progressive agenda of promoting individual autonomy over dependence, including emphasising love as the foundation for marriage instead of valuing parents' opinion, entitling women to the same civil rights enjoyed by men, encouraging the independence of children from parents, and suppressing ancestor worship. With the introduction of the one-child policy, the Chinese government aimed to improve the quality of life by decreasing the size of the population (Kipnis, 2007). Kipnis (2007) argued that overall, the government's interventions are in line with a neoliberal ideological goal of producing entrepreneurial and autonomous citizens. These interventions encourage young people to move away from their families and provide them with more flexibility in terms of how to make decisions for their own lives (Ikels, 2004).

The propaganda of the autonomous individual supports the Chinese government's modernisation project in terms of building a modern, wealthy, industrialised, and strong Chinese society. Even the economic reform of 1978 followed the 'modernisation project' pursued during the GLF and CR, that of building a modern socialist country, according to the former Chinese President and Chairman Jiang Zemin (Jiang, 1992). Various governmental agendas and national plans continue to follow the goal of this modernisation project.

Filial Piety After Economic Reform (1978)

Approaching the end of 1978, the Eleventh Central Committee of the Chinese Communist Party issued its plan for economic reform (Garnaut & Song, 2012). China transformed itself from a closed state into an open and inclusive member of the international community. Its economic policy shifted from a planned, state-owned approach to a market-oriented one that embraces globalisation (Garnaut & Song, 2012). Its economy expanded many times, to become the second biggest in the world in 2010 (Shanghai W. T. O. Affairs Consultation Centre, 2012). Industrialisation has reached unprecedented speed (Chen, 2016). According to Chen (2016), China's urbanisation rate has greatly increased, especially since the beginning of the twenty-first century. By the year 2005, the national average urbanisation rate had reached almost 43%, and it was much higher than this in economically developed provinces (Chen, 2016). The Chinese government made large financial investments in rural issues and abolished the agricultural tax in 2006 (Chen, 2016).

All the contextual changes mentioned above have been claimed as evidence of a strong neoliberal inclination (Rofel, 2007; Wu, 2010). Park (2015), writing about erosion of the norm of filial piety among Koreans, found that socio-economic changes are highly influential to the practice of filial piety. In China, after economic reform in 1978 and especially since the beginning of the twenty-first century, filial piety has been widely considered as diminishing because of neoliberalism (Nylan, 1996; Poškaitė, 2014; Xu, 2012). In the next two sections, the perceived decline of filial piety after economic reform is further discussed.

(Neoliberal) Contextual Changes in Relation to the Perceived Decline of Filial Piety

The economic reform initiated in 1978 in China has incorporated neoliberal traits that led to diminished filial practices (Chi, 2006; Rofel, 2007; Wu, 2010). Recent intergenerational research shows that adult children are more concerned with financial exchanges than emotional and spiritual (non-material) exchange (McDaniel & Zimmer, 2013). Neoliberal ideologies have been found to compromise the provision of emotional and spiritual support for aged parents in favour of financial and other types of support (Koshy, 2013). Many have argued that younger generations exercise more power than older generations in neoliberal China, and there has been a decline in children's willingness to care for their aged parents (Chen, 1996, 2009; Liu & Yuan, 2009).

Several changes in contemporary Chinese society can be related to the perceived decline in filial piety (Ikels, 2004; also Cheung & Kwan, 2009; Chi, 2006): (1) traditional large patriarchal families have been replaced by small and independent conjugal families wherein young people become attached to their conjugal family of spouse and children at the expense of the relationship with their parents and siblings; (2) rapid urbanisation, especially after the economic reform in 1978, has provided resources, benefits, and wages through market or state benefit programmes to replace family-controlled resources; and (3) public education and mass media are seen as another factor in the transformation of Chinese family values. Young people no longer need to uncritically accept the ideas of their parents, including ideas regarding how to manage intergenerational relationships.

According to Lin (2013), industrialisation and economic growth requires an ever-increasing number of cheap labourers. This has attracted peasants to work in the urban industries, as also identified by Zimmer and Kwong (2003). This migration leads to a geographical separation between migrant children and their parents, which makes the fulfilment of filial hands-on caregiving almost impossible. Lin (2013) also stated that without effective labour regulation from the government, employers exploit their employees through long working hours and little job flexibility. This makes it harder for children to meet the requirements of their employers as well as their filial obligations towards their parents.

Many scholars have noted a decline in filial piety in contemporary Chinese society. Cheung and Kwan (2009) identified social and economic trends that are challenging this ideal in China, namely those related to modernisation and industrialisation, especially urbanisation and the employment of women: 'Changed social aspirations... weaken people's acceptance of the norms of filial piety and their practice of its obligations' (Cheung & Kwan, 2009, p. 181). Liu (2012) thought the decline was due to contextual changes such as urbanisation and marketisation, which physically separate adult children from their aged parents and make it technically difficult for them to provide instrumental care. She compared urban and rural China in terms of care expectations. In urban China, following the provision of pension systems, parents' requirements of their children shifted from expecting 'care and instrumental support' to 'emotional bond and support'. By contrast, in rural areas where an adequate pension system was lacking, adult children (especially sons) continued to be expected to provide instrumental and financial care to their aged parents (Liu, 2012, p. 31).

According to Whyte and Ikels (2004), both elders and their children seem to have ambiguous feelings about the social changes caused by modernisation, and in general, elders seem to be having a difficult time because of these changes. They found that if Chinese parents and children live in the same city, practices of filial piety remain strong and effective. The situation for rural elders, however, is much bleaker. Inadequate state investment in rural health care, the consequences of the one-child policy, and the migration of children to urban areas have reduced many aged people to being burdens that their children are often unable or unwilling to provide for (Whyte & Ikels, 2004). As a consequence, older persons may experience diminished self-esteem, and suicide rates are climbing (Whyte & Ikels, 2004). Recent research by Xu (2019) claimed that around 30 per cent of Chinese older persons (including rural and urban residents) who visited the field clinics in which their research took place were victims of elder abuse. These researchers also speculated that actual levels of elder abuse and neglect might be higher, as most cases are undetected and unreported due to the cultural norm of prioritising the preservation of honour and harmony.

Neoliberalism as Culprit?

Another aspect of Chinese neoliberalism is a sense of insecurity about the future, which is also linked to the decline of filial piety. According to Foucault (2008), neoliberalism results in the reconceptualisation of labour from a fixed and abstract entity to a set of skills and attributes that enable an individual to earn money over a lifetime. Insufficient job opportunities generated by a non-state-regulated market and urbanisation have created a sense of insecurity among young people. For example, according to Miller (2004), due to financial pressures and insecurity about the future, many daughters-in-law no longer have the option to be housewives and to care for their parents-in-law and children. According to Koshy (2013), to cope with this insecurity, the parent generation has redefined child-rearing so that rather than seeing their children as their future caregivers, they value cultivating their children's employment-related skills as sources of future income. Moreover, a lack of an efficient and effective social welfare system deepens the sense of insecurity felt by the parent generation. Children are valued as old-age risk insurance, which reflects on a traditional term, *yan er wei fang lao* (养儿为防老, child-rearing is for old age). Recently, researchers such as S. Chen (2009) have claimed that parents, especially those who only have one child, tend to invest an increasingly greater proportion of their financial assets into their child's education and on marriage expenses. Moreover, according to Huang and Lin (2018), adult children also draw on support from parents to meet their childcare, laundry, food preparation, housing purchase, and other needs; this is especially evident in migrant workers' families. Thus intergenerational relationships are therefore centred on heavy parental investment in their children's education, marriage, and training for the labour market, as well as caring for grandchildren to support the pursuit of employment (Chen, 1996; Chen et al., 2011; Ikels, 2006).

It is understandable that researchers have blamed neoliberalisation for the perceived decline in filial care. It is undeniable that neoliberal marketisation and industrialisation have had impacts on filial family relationships and filial practices. However, neoliberalism might not be the sole culprit in the decline. In the Chinese context, it is too simplistic to solely blame neoliberal marketisation after economic reform in 1978 for the diminishment of filial piety.

The Government's Response to Claims of Diminishing Filial Piety: Re-Embracing Chinese Traditional Cultural Norms and the Parent-Visiting Law

Over the last few years, the Chinese government has countered the claim that neoliberal social transformation has undermined filial practices and perceptions by deploying propaganda and laws to facilitate filial piety.

Propaganda to Revive Chinese Traditional Culture and the *Guoxue* Movement. In the sixth Plenary Session of the Seventeenth Central Committee in 2011, a bill was passed labelled 'Decision of the CPC Central Committee on major issues pertaining to deepening reforms of the cultural system and promoting the great development and flourishing of socialist culture' (Ouyang & Cui, 2013). The Central Committee emphasised that Chinese culture, as *yuanyuanliuchang* (源远流长, long-standing and well established) and *bodajingshen* (博大进深, broad and profound), provides non-material assets for the people and also contributes to the development of human civilisation (Ouyang & Cui, 2013). According to Ouyang and Cui (2013), the governmental discourse has recently begun to reflect the importance of Chinese traditional culture and values. These authors expressed their expectation that Chinese society would re-embrace the superiority of traditional values as the government deepens its acknowledgement of traditional culture and values. In the 2016 Two Sessions (the annual sessions of China's top legislative and advisory bodies), a draft Law of Protection of Ethnic and Folk Traditional Culture was submitted to the Central Committee (posted on the official website of the National People's Congress of the People's Republic of China; Zhang, 2016). There have also already been actions to protect traditional ethnic and folk culture in civil society, for example through intellectual property laws (Guan, 2005).

The government is not alone in endeavouring to propel these social and cultural movements, as the academic world and wider society have also supported this return to valuing traditional Chineseness. Interest in *guoxue* (国学, studies in Chinese ancient civilisation such as philosophy, arts, history, and archaeology) is on the rise among scholars and the general public (Song, 2015). This, together with the New Confucianism movement, resonates with the governmental agenda of promoting Chinese traditional culture and virtues. Both *guoxue* and New Confucianism have received criticism on the part of scholars such as Song Zhimin for bringing back too many ideals rooted in Confucian traditional morality with insufficient critique and a lack of adaptation to the current Chinese context (Song, 2015). The propaganda for reviving Chinese traditional culture contradicts the modernisation project, which was determined to eradicate traditional culture and philosophy during the CR.

The 'Parent-Visiting Law'. The government has played an important role in supporting movements promoting filial piety, as discussed above (Ouyang & Cui, 2013). The Chinese government issued a 2012 revision of the Law on the Protection of the Rights and Interests of the Elderly (中华人民共和国 老年人权益保障法, 2012修订) to legally oblige adult children to visit parents. This revision came into effect on 1 July 2013 (during the proposal stage of my PhD; *Asian News International*, 2013). According to the law, adult children who fail to comply with visiting requirements can face legal charges and other penalities, and senior parents are able to sue their children for not visiting them (Fan, 2013). The law has received criticism since its enactment, both domestically and internationally. According to Makinen (2013), compliance with this law would be difficult for migrant peasant workers, especially if they are only children. Moreover, the frequency with which children should visit their parents cannot be easily quantified (Gruijters, 2017; MacLeod, 2013).

Evolving Nature of Filial Piety and Lack of Historical (Genealogical) Analysis during the Great Leap Forward and Cultural Revolution. Filial piety itself has been constantly shaped and (re)constructed by various social and political forces over time. As shown in the discussion of its historical trajectory, filial piety has been through several different stages in the past 2,000–3,000 years, and it has been used by the ruling class and embedded into people's everyday lives in unique ways at each stage. According to Luo (2013), this deeply accepted and practised cultural way of being was heavily criticised throughout the twentieth century by scholars and in political discourse. The historical trajectories of filial piety demonstrate that economic reform is not the only force that reframed or changed filial perceptions for Chinese people.

According to Z. Zhao (2017), studies of filial piety after economic reform have mostly focused on analysing the social construction of filial piety in the dynastic period. Criticism concerning filial piety during the New Culture Movement (1910s–1920s) can be found too. However, there is a lack of literature on the trajectory of filial piety between the foundation of the People's Republic of China and the initiation of economic reform in 1978, symbolised by the GLF in 1950s and the CR from 1966 to 1976, as well as early in the economic reform, from the late 1970s to the 1980s. Z. Zhao (2017) briefly mentioned that he did not find any articles published about filial piety before 1984, for obvious reasons. According to Wang (2014), there was a period of time during which filial piety was heavily tampered with, especially during the CR. According to Xu (2007) and Leese (2011), the GLF and the CR together constitute a period of trauma that is considered to be a taboo topic in the Chinese political and public discourse. A more thorough historical analysis is required in an investigation of current discourses of filial piety, and I pursue this in subsequent chapters, including in analysing the accounts of my participants.

Conclusion

According to Ikels (2004), filial piety becomes a practical exchange in rural areas in contemporary China rather than a cultural and moral norm and ideal for people to follow and cultivate. Many scholars claimed that after economic reform in 1978, filial piety was diminished by the neoliberal modernisation project (e.g., Cheung & Kwan, 2009; Ikels, 2004; Koshy, 2013; Nylan, 1996; Poškaitė, 2014; Wang, 2016; Xu, 2012). In the wake of such diminishing, the Chinese government has encouraged family care and promoted the cultural value of filial piety (McDaniel & Zimmer, 2013). The historical trajectory of filial piety indicates, however, that the decline in filial piety (or neo-Confucian filial discourse) started much earlier than economic reform. During the New Culture Movement, GLF, and CR, filial piety, along with (neo-)Confucianism, was heavily criticised and attempted to be discarded altogether. Thus, the contemporary discourse of filial piety is complex, and this complexity needs to be understood and addressed.

References

Ames, R. T., & Rosemont, Jr, H. (2010). *The analects of Confucius: A philosophical translation*. Ballantine.

Asian News International. (2013, July 1). China passes law forcing kids to visit elderly parents.

Bachman, D. (2006). *Bureaucracy, economy, and leadership in China: The institutional origins of the Great Leap Forward*. Cambridge University Press.

Chen, F., Liu, G., & Mair, C. A. (2011). Intergenerational ties in context: Grandparents caring for grandchildren in China. *Social Forces, 90*(2), 571–594. https://doi.org/10.1093/sf/sor012

Chen, J. (1996). *Old age support and intergenerational relations in urban China: Maintenance of obligations between older parents and children*. Doctoral dissertation, The University of Michigan, Ann Arbor.

Chen, J. G. (2016). *Economic development and reform deepening in China*. Taylor and Francis.

Chen, K. (2002). *Research on Confucius thought*孔子思想研究. *People's Daily* 人民日报出版社.

Chen, S. (2009). Aging with Chinese characteristics: A public policy perspective. *Ageing International, 34*(3), 172–188. https://doi.org/10.1007/s12126-009-9043-6

Cheung, C. K., & Kwan, A. Y.-H. (2009). The erosion of filial piety by modernisation in Chinese cities. *Ageing & Society, 29*(2), 179–198. https://doi.org/10.1017/S0144686X08007836

Chi, L. K. (2006). Untimely reflections on modernization in China. *Peripherie, 26*(103), 255–290.

Fan, F. (2013, July 2). Parent-visiting services offered in wake of law. *People*. http://en.people.cn

Feng, Y. (1995). *History of Chinese philosophy*中国哲学史. Zhonghua Shuju.

"Neo-Confucianism". (2016, April 11). *Neo-Confucianism*. http://faculty.washington.edu/mkalton/NeoConfucianism.htm

Foster, R. (2014). *Neo-Confucianism*. Oxford University Press.

Foucault, M. (1970). *The archaeology of knowledge*. Tavistock.

Foucault, M. (2008). *The birth of biopolitics*. Trans. G. Burchell. Palgrave Macmillan

Garnaut, R., & Song, L. (2012). *China: Twenty years of economic reform*. ANU Press.

Ge, X. (2016). A tale of "*ku*" (bitter) v.s. "*tian*" (sweet): Understanding China's "*yiku sitian*" movement in the 1960s and 1970s from the perspective of cultural discourse analysis. Doctoral dissertation, University of Massachusetts.

Goldin, P. R. (2011). *Confucianism*. Acumen.

Gruijters, R. J. (2017). Intergenerational contact in Chinese families: Structural and cultural explanations. *Journal of Marriage and Family, 79*(3), 758–768. https://doi.org/10.1111/jomf.12390

Guan, Y. (2005). Legal protection for traditional knowledge and traditional culture expressions "传统知识及传统文化表达的法律保护问题". *Normal University of Guizhou University Press (Social Science Session), 2*(3), 14–26. http://www.gznu.edu.cn

Huang, C., & Lin, J. (2018). Intergenerational financial support exchange between adult children and baby boomer parents: The impact of life events

成年子女与婴儿潮世代父母的代间经济支持交换:生命事件的影响. *Journal of Human Development and Family 人类发展与家庭学报, 19*, 15–43.

Ikels, C. (2004). *Filial piety: Practice and discourse in contemporary East Asia*. Stanford University Press.

Ikels, C. (2006). Economic reform and intergenerational relationships in China. *Oxford Development Studies, 34*(4), 387–400. https://doi.org/10.1080/13600810601045619

Ji, F. (2004). *Linguistic engineering: Language and politics in Mao's China*. University of Hawai'i Press.

Jiang, Z. (1992). Speed up economic reform and modernisation construction for bigger success in obtaining socialism with Chinese characteristics 加快改革开放和现代化建设步伐夺取有中国特色社会主义事业的更大胜利——在中国共产党第十四次全国代表大会上的报告. *Qianxian 前线, Z1*, 5–22.

Li, J., & Nie, H. (2012). Confucian filial piety, economic growth and divergence among civilizations. *Chinese Social Science (English Version)中国社会科学: 英文版, 33*(4), 69–88. https://doi.org/10.1080/02529203.2012.731802

Kipnis, A. (2007). Neoliberalism reified: Suzhi discourse and tropes of neoliberalism in the People's Republic of China. *Journal of the Royal Anthropological Institute, 13*(2), 383–400. https://doi.org/10.1111/j.1467-9655.2007.00432.x

Koshy, S. (2013). Neoliberal family matters. *American Literary History, 25*(2), 344–380. https://doi.org/10.1093/alh/ajt006

Kraus, R. C. (2012). *The cultural revolution: A very short introduction*. Oxford University Press.

Leese, D. (2011). *Mao cult: Rhetoric and ritual in China's cultural revolution*. Cambridge University Press.

Li, H. (2014). Chinese traditional filial piety and its modern significance 中国传统孝道及其现代价值. *Technology Prospect 科技展望, 20*, 238–45. http://www.zxqyzz.com

Li, J. (2003). The core of Confucian learning. *American Psychologist, 58*(2), 146–147. https://doi.org/10.1037/0003-066X.58.2.146

Li, R. (2004). Power and humanity: A study of public canteens during the Great Leap Forward 权力与人性: 大跃进时期公共食堂研究. *Open Times 开放时代, 1*, 009. http://tongtor.cqbgbk.com/index.html

Li, X. (2003). Investigation and discussion of the May 4th and new culture movements in relation to culture and tradition 五四新文化运动与民族文化传统关系问题再探讨. *Teaching and Research 教学与研究, 4*. http://tongtor.cqbgbk.com/index.html

Lin, X. (2013). *Gender, modernity and male migrant workers in China: Becoming a "modern" man*. Routledge.

Ling, L. (1994). Rationalizations for state violence in Chinese politics: The hegemony of parental governance. *Journal of Peace Research, 31*(4), 393–405. https://doi.org/10.1177/0022343394031004003

Liu, L., & Yuan, C. (2009). Construction of palliative care training contents in China: A Delphi study. *Cancer Nursing, 32*(6), 446–455. https://doi.org/10.1097/NCC.0b013e3181ab572e

Liu, W. (2012). The diminishing of filial piety? The perception, behaviour, and relevant affecting factors of adult children caring for aged parents 孝道衰落? 成年子女支持父母的观念, 行为及其影响因素. *Youth Research 青年研究, 2*, 22–32. http://www.zhazhi.com/qikan/shxzx/shx/1355.html

Liu, Z. (2013). The contention of "a hundred schools of thought" and development of the theory of monarchism during the Warring States period. *Contemporary Chinese Thought, 45*(2–3), 32–54. https://doi.org/10.2753/CSP1097-1467450202

Luk, M. Y. L. (1989). Review of the book *The Chinese enlightenment: Intellectuals and the legacy of the May Fourth movement of 1919*, by V. Schwarcz. *The China Quarterly, 117*, 155–56. https://doi.org/10.1017/S0305741000023754

Luo, C. (2013). *Filial piety and its "tianjingdiyi" 天经地义论孝道*. Guang Ming Ri Bao 光明日报出版社.

Luo, M., & Wang, S. (2013). *Filial laws and assizes in every dynasty*. Guang Ming Ri Bao 光明日报出版社.

MacFarquhar, R., & Mao, Z. (1989). *The secret speeches of Chairman Mao: From the Hundred Fowers to the Great Leap Forward*. Council on East Asian Studies/Harvard University.

MacLeod, C. (2013, August 8). China orders children to visit their aging parents: Law allows lawsuits against offspring for money and visitation. *USA Today*.

Makinen, J. (2013, August 30). China's "visit your parents" law weighs on many in one-child nation. *Pittsburgh Post-Gazette*.

Manning, K. E., & Wemheuer, F. (2011). *Eating bitterness: New perspectives on China's Great Leap Forward and famine*. UBC Press.

McDaniel, S., & Zimmer, Z. (2013). *Global ageing in the 21st Century: Challenges, opportunities and implications*. Ashgate.

Miller, E. T. (2004). Filial daughters, filial sons: Comparisons from rural north China. In C. Ikels (Ed.), *Filial piety: Practice and discourse in contemporary East Asia* (pp. 34–52). Stanford University Press.

Mufson, S. (1996). Maoism, Confucianism blur into nationalism series: Asia's dragon: What is Chinese nationalism? *The Washington Post, 1*(3), 1–12.

Nylan, M. (1996). Confucian piety and individualism in Han China. *Journal of the American Oriental Society, 116*(1), 1–27. https://doi.org/10.2307/606369

Ouyang, J., & Cui, C. (2013). The cultivation of Chinese traditonal culture and socialist core value perceptions "中国传统文化与社会主义核心价值观的培育". *Shandong Social Science 山东社会科学, 3*, 11–15. http://www.sdshkx.com/

Park, H. (2015). Legislating for filial piety: An indirect approach to promoting family support and responsibility for older people in Korea. *Journal of Aging & Social Policy, 27*(3), 280–293. https://doi.org/10.1080/08959420.2015.1024536

Peng, X. (1987). Demographic consequences of the Great Leap Forward in China's provinces. *Population and Development Review, 13*(4), 639–70. https://onlinelibrary.wiley.com/journal/17284457

Poškaitė, L. (2014). Filial piety (xiao 孝) for the contemporary and global world. *Asian Studies, 2*(1), 99–114. https://doi.org/10.4312/as.2014.2.1.99-114

Rofel, L. (2007). *Desiring China: Experiments in neoliberalism, sexuality, and public culture*. Duke University Press.

Rosen, S. (2007). *Mao's last revolution*. Harvard University Press.

Shanghai World Trade Organisation Affairs Consultation Centre. (2012). *2011 China's trade performance report: World economy restructuring and China's trade*. SCPG.

Song, Z. (2015). From "accordingly" to "expanding": To discuss Feng Youlan's new thoughts on Confucianism 从"照着讲"到"接着讲"——论冯友兰讲儒学的新思路. *Social Science Frontline*, (2), 9–16.

St. André, J. . (2018). Consequences of the conflation of *xiao* and filial piety in English. *Translation and Interpreting Studies, 13*(2), 293–316. https://doi.org/10.1075/tis.00017.sta

Tang, B., & Li, C. (2001). An analysis of Confucianist filial piety in ancient China. *Hunan Normal University Social Science 5*, 223–28. http://skc.hunnu.edu.cn/

Trnka, S., & Trundle, C. (2014). Competing responsibilities: Moving beyond neoliberal responsibilisation. *Anthropological Forum, 24*(2), 136–153. https://doi.org/10.1080/00664677.2013.879051

Wang, D. (2010). *The fall of humanity 人类的没落*. Xianxi People's Publisher.

Wang, D. (2016). The one with no fear has a heart of fear: Three fears of junzi and its educational purpose for youth 无畏者怀有的敬畏之心——君子三畏及对青年的借鉴意义. *Social Science 社会科学:全文版* (12), 00047. http://www.cqvip.com/QK/72177X/

Wang, Y. (2014). *Chinese traditional filial piety and contemporary rural family elder care research 中国传统孝道思想与当代农村家庭养老研究*. QingHai Normal University 青海师范大学.

Whyte, M. K., & Ikels, C. (2004). Filial obligations in Chinese families: Paradoxes of modernization. In C. Ikels (Ed.), *Filial piety: Practice and discourse in contemporary East Asia* (pp. 106–127). Stanford University Press.

Wu, F. (2010). How neoliberal is China's reform? The origins of change during transition. *Eurasian Geography and Economics, 51*(5), 619–631. https://doi.org/10.2747/1539-7216.51.5.619

Wu, G. (2012). *China 1966–1976, Cultural revolution revisited: Can it happen again?* Novinka.

Wu, L. (2013). Cultural Revolution (China). In D. A. Snow, D. Della Porta, B. Klandermans, & D. McAdam (Eds.), *The Wiley-Blackwell encyclopedia of social and political movements*. Wiley-Blackwell. https://doi.org/10.1002/9780470674871.wbespm270

Xi, X., & Jin, C. (2006). *Brief history of the "Cultural Revolution" "文化大革命"简史*. CCP History Republisher 中共党史出版社.

Xu, F. (2007). The traumatic memory of anti-rightism 50 years later 五十年后的"反右"创伤记忆. *Contemporary Chinese Research, 3*, 98.

Xu, J. (2012). Filial piety and intergenerational communication in China: A nationwide study. *Journal of International Communication, 18*(1), 33–48. https://doi.org/10.1080/13216597.2012.662466

Xu, J. (2019). Elder abuse and mental health: The moderating effect of social support 老年人虐待与心理健康:社会支持的调节效应. *Journal of Chinese Disease Control 中华疾病控制杂志* (11), 1323–27.

Yan, J. (1999). Evaluation of the argument between "4th May", "Cultural Revolution" and the traditional culture 评"五四","文革"与传统文化的论争. *Chinese and Foreign Culture and Discussion 中外文化与文论, 1*(2), 2–13.

You, J. (2006). The Li School's betrayal of Confucianism from the perspective of *sangang wuchang* 从"三纲五常"看程朱理学对孔孟儒学的背叛. *Ezhou University Paper 鄂州大学学报, 13*(1), 57–59. http://xuebao.ezutsg.cn/

Zhang, G. (2009). Taoist filial thought research 道家孝道思想研究. *Yuxi Normal College Journal 玉溪师范学院学报* (2), 10–15. http://xuebao.yxnu.net/

Zhang, J. (2016). The formation of the *Book of Filial Piety* and its significance《孝经》的形成及历史意义. *Yilinwenhui 意林文汇* (20), 60–78. http://mall.cnki.net/magazine/magalist/YKWH.htm

Zhang, X. (2017). Mainland contemporary neo-Confucianists and neo-Kangyouweiism 大陆新儒家与新康有为主义的兴起. *Cultural Aspect 文化纵横* (3), 98–107. http://www.21bcr.com/

Zhao, Z. (2017). Research review of filial culture since economic reform 改革开放以来孝文化研究述评. *Xihua University Scholarly (Philosophy and Social Science) 西华大学学报 (哲学社会科学版), 5*, 003. http://qk.xhu.edu.cn/1908/list.htm

Zhu, S. (1999). Li School's abstinence and its negative influence 略论理学禁欲主义思想的形成及其负面影响. *Qi Lu Scholarly 齐鲁学刊* (4), 60–64. http://qlxk2003.toug.com.cn/

Zimmer, Z., & Kwong, J. (2003). Family size and support of older adults in urban and rural China: Current effects and future implications. *Demography, 40*(1), 23–44. https://doi.org/10.1353/dem.2003.0010

CHAPTER 3

Research on Care and Filial Piety in China and Lack of 'Localised' Theoretical Grounding

Introduction

Following on from the discussion in previous chapters of a flawed perception of neoliberalism as the sole or primary culprit behind a decline in filial piety in China, this chapter identifies a gap in the literature in terms of the complex impacts of socio-economic changes after economic reform on migrant peasant workers caring for their parents. Considerations of care behaviours and filial piety are often conflated, and this conflation is related to claims about the relationship between neoliberalism and the decline of filial piety. Therefore, the relationship between filial piety and care calls for deeper analysis. A review of the literature also shows other significant gaps, including the infrequency of migrant peasant workers as research subjects and the lack of qualitative studies.

In the next section, I review recent studies that examine the relationship between modernisation theory and filial piety, work on theories of intergenerational relationships, and Chinese filial piety studies, including studies that employ discourse analysis. I include literature relevant to building the foundation for my comprehensive methodology which involves a Foucauldian discourse analysis that is culturally integrated with Chineseness. This lays the ground for the methodological innovation section in which I explain how my research addresses an age-old question: how should/could a western methodology be adapted to a specific cultural issue in the east?

L. He, *Care Work, Migrant Peasant Families and Discourse of Filial Piety in China*, https://doi.org/10.1007/978-981-16-1880-2_3

A Review of Existing Research on Filial Care

In this section, I focus on previous work that is specifically relevant to care (provided by adult children to aged parents) and filial piety and I identify the features of that work.

Care and the Concept of Filial Piety in Relation to Care

According to Z. Zhao (2017), there have been approximately 3,000 studies published on filial piety between 1978 and 2015 in China. He found that research interest in filial culture has increased rapidly, shown by a rise in publications on the topic from zero articles in 1984 to almost 300 in 2015, and identified a research focus on filial piety in relation to political policy and legislation. However, despite the increasing quantity of publications, there remains a serious lack of research on certain aspects of filial piety, such as health and care.

In the existing literature on filial piety and care experiences, many researchers conflate care provided by adult children to their aged parents with filial care and filial piety. Traditionally, providing care for parents was the foremost component of filial piety (Liu & Yu, 2008), and it continues to be regarded as the most important criterion for being filial (Q. Zhao, 2017). Lu (2016) considered adult children's caregiving for parents as a direct embodiment of filial piety. Other researchers, such as Wen (2017), have also attributed the provision of care (including instrumental, material, and non-material care) to filial piety. However, some scholars, such as Wei and Zhong (2016) and Huang (2006), following the western (and more general global) research approach, discussed filial piety as an important cultural motive for providing care to aged parents, along with other factors (e.g., intergenerational exchange, community negotiation, and socio-economic structural constraints). Overall, however, there has not been much research into the motives for providing care for aged parents in China and how caregivers discursively construct their care experiences. Huang (2006) conducted research into various mechanisms for encouraging caregiving behaviours for aged parents, such as setting an example for the next generation, intergenerational exchange, traditional filial perceptions, community and extended family persuasion, and notions of repayment of favours (the children feel they need to repay their parents, and they do so by taking care of them when their parents are old). The latter mechanism reflects the concept of *yang er wei fang lao*养儿为防

老—to raise children as a safety net for old age. All the factors/motives in Huang's (2006) research can also be seen as components of filial discourse.

Recent socio-economic structural change has presented new challenges for migrant peasant workers to provide the same level of care for parents as they used to, according to Wen (2017). A simplistic conflation of caregiving for aged parents with filial piety can result in the assumption that a decline in care behaviours equates to a decline of filial piety. However, according to Liu (2012), adherence to the ideal of filial piety itself has not diminished. She claimed that the aspect of obedience to parents that was embedded in neo-Confucian discourses of filial piety has significantly declined, but there did appear to be a decline in the provision of instrumental care for aged parents in rural areas. Her research showed the willingness to provide care and to be filial to parents remained very strong.

Some Chinese researchers have investigated filial piety as a means of resolving eldercare issues, yet without exploring the mechanism of care relationships between parents and children. Xiao (2000) contended that filial piety is essential for Chinese eldercare whether in ancient or contemporary society. According to Zhu and Liang (2006), filial piety is the realistic choice for rural eldercare in contemporary Chinese society. Pan et al. (2006) agreed that Confucian ethics of filial piety continues to retain its importance and remains a positive influence on rural family relationships and caregiving. However, most of these scholars argued that the mode of rural eldercare will need to adopt an aspect of social institutional care in the future. These researchers tend to consider filial piety as a concrete resource (such as a well-established pension system would be) that can be called upon and used to deliver services, without seeming to properly understand what filial piety means or encompasses for Chinese people in current Chinese society.

Lack of Qualitative Data

Much research on filial care has tended to adopt quantitative methodologies to gather statistical and other quantifiable data. In the research of Gruijters (2017), Lai (2010), and Cheung and Kwan (2009), filial piety was studied through different informal care variables, using statistical formulas to test hypotheses of filial piety. Sun (2002) claimed that Chinese sociological research is still dominated by quantitative methods such as questionnaires. Lum et al. (2016) adopted an approach using large questionnaire surveys, which consisted of numerous 5-point Likert-type questions, to test existing tools that are purported to identify the level of people's filial piety, such as the Formal Filial Piety Scale. Scholars who deem filial piety to be beneficial (applying a functionalist model) in contemporary Chinese society as well as scholars who deem it to be harmful (applying a conflict model) have tended to adopt quantitative methodologies and data to justify their hypotheses. For example, Lee (1997) used a questionnaire to compare the functional role of filial piety in fostering family harmony and intergenerational solidarity among people in several cities. On the other hand, Ho (1994) used questionnaires to test the hypothesis that filial piety contains an authoritarian morality, correlates with parents' high emphasis on obedience, and can negatively affect children's self-development.

According to Hooyman and Kiyak (2008), internationally there has been increasing adoption of qualitative methodologies in social research in recent years. However, in the Chinese context, research on intergenerational relationships and eldercare has mainly focused on quantitative data and analysis (Hooyman & Kiyak, 2008). In a caregiving context, it is understandable that practitioners, managers, and policymakers wish to quantify care tasks, time spent on care, and other resource requirements. However, in a context of exploring how people make sense of cultural norms and feelings, it can be problematic to use a quantitative sociological approach. Alasuutari (1995) stated that there is no universal 'truth' within culture studies and held that culture should be studied through subjectivity but not through hierarchy (Alasuutari, 1995). Quantitative approaches that value hierarchical data and the testing of hypotheses, by contrast, suggest that there are cultural realities to be uncovered and that there are meaningful answers to questions such as: How much care does a child need to give before they can be considered as filial? How often does a migrant peasant worker need to come home to be filial? More researchers have come to realise that changing social contexts and fluid nature of filial perception makes it difficult to use a quantitative approach to define filial piety simplistically and that there is a need for more complex explorations. As Willig (2001) also noted, qualitative research focuses on how people make sense of their cultural world mostly through unmeasurable means, and how subjectivity is constructed in the process.

As Jones (1985) wrote:

> [T]o understand other persons' constructions of reality we would do well to ask them... and to ask them in such a way that they can tell us in their terms (rather than those imposed rigidly and *a priori* by ourselves) and in a depth which addresses the rich context that is the substance of their meanings. (Jones, 1985, p. 56)

Qualitative techniques allow space for accessing people's understandings and perceptions. According to Punch (2005), these techniques also allow different world views to come together. In quantitative research, such 'chaotic' differentiation is often not accepted; rather, views and answers are simplified to accommodate the predetermined hypothesis or 'truth' (Punch, 2005).

Since the end of the last century, qualitative research has become increasingly popular in health care, due to its flexibility in research methods and approaches to analysis (Pope et al., 2000). Sun (2002) claimed that qualitative methodology such as discourse analysis can provide deep insight into certain social phenomena. Contemporary Chinese society is experiencing a massive scale of social transformation, and the research methodology and analysis should be able to reflect the complexity of such transformation. Even though quantitative methodological data has its own merits, qualitative approaches with a deeper investigation into the hidden mechanisms behind certain social phenomena are more suitable. Subjective data enables researchers to delve deep into social phenomena and detect various hidden or taken for granted processes.

Limited Literature on Caregivers and Migrant Peasant Workers as Caregivers

Migrant peasant workers are a social group that is particularly strongly affected by neoliberal marketisation and urbanisation in China. The distance between their residential location and that of their parents, as well as other factors (such as their marginalised social status and lack of access to unpaid leave to enable them to provide parental care), makes migrant peasant workers highly susceptible to changes in filial practices and perceptions. According to Ikels (2004), migrant peasant workers remain the main care source for rural elders. It is important to investigate the mechanisms of the caregiving practices and perceptions for the sake of rural elders' health safety net and quality of life.

Family care is an indispensable resource in China, where social institutions for aged care are not as established as in many other countries (Chen & Hu, 2015). But despite the important role they play, informal caregivers who provide home-based care to elderly patients have been an underserved and underresearched group whose existence has only not long ago entered the cultural and literary consciousness in China (Li et al., 2009; Zhu et al., 2019). Even more so than in the west, despite the important roles informal caregivers play in caring for patients and their experiences have only recently begun to be considered (Xiao et al., 2014). According to Li and Zhao (2009), the importance of family care itself is now emerging as a topic of concern for both the Chinese government and Chinese academia.

There is little research that has investigated how adult children make subjective sense of their caring experiences through the discourse of filial piety, nor how adult children who are caregivers are affected by changes that have taken place after economic reform. It is not difficult to locate research that suggests a decline in filial piety has led to changes in care patterns and other social phenomena, such as an increasing rate of elder suicide (Ikels, 2004). Much research has focused on the health conditions of elderly parents and the care they receive, and the relationship of these factors to the perceived erosion of filial piety (Ding, 2003; Liu, 2012; Lu, 2016; Liu & Yu, 2008; Wen, 2017; Q. Zhao, 2017; Zhong & He, 2014). Few researchers have focused on migrant peasant workers' subjective perceptions of filial piety and filial practices, and only a few Chinese scholars (e.g., Lin, 2013) have examined the subjective construction of the filial self in relation to the contextual changes in these workers' lives. Lin (2013) interviewed male migrant peasant workers and found that they used filial piety as a mechanism to make sense of their self-identity in a modern city. Filial piety was deemed to be a positive cultural resource that migrant peasant workers could rely on when they were facing marginalised and deprived social circumstances. Kuo and Tsou (2016) discovered that filial piety could also act as an obstacle for children to ask for help or make use of institutional care assistance even when this exists in a modernised society. Clearly, children's subjective construction of the filial self in relation to social and economic changes needs to be examined more thoroughly and directly. Such an examination should include an exploration of the impact of contextual changes after economic reform on migrant peasant workers.

The literature conveys a somewhat underarticulated but nevertheless evident social and theoretical assumption that if migrant peasants' traditionally strongly engrained filial practices and perceptions can change, other demographic groups may also change their relationship to filial piety. Qualitative research, compared to quantitative research, can lead to more nuanced understandings of reflexive discursive constructions of filial piety and caregiving, and can help to avoid overgeneralising inferences to other Chinese social groups drawn from a heretofore relatively minimal understanding of migrant peasant workers' care experiences. Awareness of the need for more nuanced understanding may lead to more appropriate research that is able to capture the complex needs of other demographic groups and ultimately lead to better and more tailored policy responses.

Lack of Historical (Genealogical) Analysis During the Great Leap Forward and the Cultural Revolution

According to Zhou et al. (2016) and Ji (2009), in recent years work on filial piety has predominantly focused on ancient texts relating to filial piety. New Confucian scholars (introduced in Chapter 2) have tended to investigate the origins of filial piety and how it was practised in dynastic periods of China. For instance, Zhang's (2000) research paper 'The Formation and Evolution of Confucian Filial Piety' comprehensively discussed how the Confucian filial perspective was formed and how this evolved through Chinese history (until the last dynasty). Zeng (2002) articulated the historical path of filial piety and touched upon the variations of filial discourse that developed since the Qin (221–207 BCE) and Han (202 BCE–220 CE) dynasties. The book *Selected Writings on Chinese Ancient Filial Piety*, edited by Luo (2003), focused on the construct of filial discourse in the academic, social, and political scopes, and laws and assizes in every Chinese dynasty.

The existing literature has largely ignored that there was a time during the Great Leap Forward (GLF) and the Cultural Revolution (CR) when children rebelled against their parents and filial piety was heavily criticised by both the government and the public (Wang, 2014). After economic reform, memories and documents relating to the critique of filial piety that occurred during the 1950s and between 1966 and 1976 appeared to become 'forgotten' and lost from private and public records. According to Fan (2007), filial piety enables the state to be excused from social care responsibilities. The time of the GLF and the CR was often referred to vaguely as 'those years' by my participants.

Theoretical Developments Around Filial Piety

Next follows a more in-depth review of trends in the literature that helps to establish the need for my research theoretically, both reflecting problematic aspects of past research projects and identifying forms of inquiry that may prove more powerful and compelling.

Modernisation Theory and Filial Piety

Perhaps one of the most prevalent social theoretical bases applied in research on filial piety has to do with modernisation theory, that is to say the contextualisation of filial piety issues within the ongoing demographic, economic, and political changes associated with China's post-reform economic acceleration. Ikels (2006) provided an overview of the ways that modernisation theory is being applied to issues related to filial piety in China. She 'examine[d] the impact of post-Mao economic reform... on the support systems of China's elderly' (Ikels, 2006, p. 387). As she noted (p. 388), 'modernisation theory prioritises economic change' and tends to lead to fairly high-level findings that are uniformly grim for the rural elders, as traditional forms of employment and support for rural elders are undermined by industrialisation and urbanisation. While these formulations 'tend to predict a more or less uniform course and set of outcomes' (p. 388), a specific east Asian regional application of modernisation theory was based on the notion that either Confucian values, or more empirically, 'high rates of intergenerational co-residence, high rates of continued employment of older people, etc.' could mitigate these consequences for Chinese rural elders (p. 388).

As discussed earlier in this chapter, most sociological literature relating to China appears to be fairly pessimistic on the question of whether the various institutions of elder support related to filial piety remain intact despite the changes associated with modernisation. According to Ikels (2006, p. 397), the 'consequences of modernisation' are likely to be 'especially severe' for aged Chinese because of the 'reversed sequencing of the historical process'. The institutions of care for rural elders were based on rural social and family patterns, including big families where children remain in proximity to their parents, but the contextual trend is from a rural to an urban economy and towards one-child families. The demographic pattern typical of developing countries like China is that an economic boom precedes a delayed decline in fertility over an extended period of time (spanning years), allowing a transitional rural generation to receive support from families that are still relatively large. Moreover, China's accelerated industrial development, in association with a massive level of urbanisation and combined with its one-child policy, have begun to make their impacts felt and have created extreme pressure on the current generation of young people who are struggling to support their parents. Ikels (2006) thought that these trends are too powerful for Confucian values and filial piety to resist, despite the best intentions of the children of rural elders.

Ikels's (2006) study pointed to concrete and pragmatic policy reforms that can mitigate the worst consequences of modernisation for rural older persons as well as the burdens of filial support that are facing their children. These include new insurance programmes, better health funding, better training of home care workers, programmes to assist older persons in socialising outside of the home and being more engaged in civic society, and other approaches to 'develop ways of financially supporting the rural elderly' (Ikels, 2006, p. 397). These solutions seem to follow from assumptions about how western modernisation processes map to changes in household resources, rather than into any deep connection with what Chinese rural elders want, need, and ask for from their families. Although it is Ikels's intention to reassure young people, her statement in fact indicates that adult children are still embracing the concept of filial piety and are highly willing to provide care to parents, in contradiction to the perception of modernisation theory about the decline of filial piety.

The analysis provided by modernisation theory, however deliberate, empirical, and sound it might appear, seems not so much to diagnose and solve a problem in a particular context as to point to a set of frustrations in line with a western modernisation path. The solutions proposed are other than reflexive, but perhaps idealistic. It would seem more helpful to develop a more refined and contextualised picture of the concrete and subjective ways that people are engaging in the struggle to support their parents, and of how they themselves understand the challenges they face and how they attempt to overcome those. Such an analysis (which I pursued through a Foucauldian discourse analysis) should be more open to surprising insights based on subjective perceptions rather than reified theoretical variables predicted by modernisation theory. Such a discursive analysis might lead to deeper pragmatic advice for other people engaged in the same or a similar struggle. It could also generate more innovative policy thinking aimed at achieving effective change, or at least provide an empathetic and consolatory narrative for the individuals involved in the Chinese context. A discursive analysis on the topic of filial piety in this research might reposition modernisation theory as the context for a more discursive analysis of the phenomenon of filial piety in current Chinese society. In fact Ikels herself followed the discursive analytical path in editing the 2004 collection of essays *Practice and Discourse in Contemporary East Asia* (Ikels, 2004).

Theories on Intergenerational Relationships

There is a well-established body of literature theorising intergenerational relationships. According to Liou (2011), as the most basic relationship in human society, the intergenerational relationship captures the various modes of relations that emerge between generations through, for example, resource sharing and emotional communication.

Some researchers adopt social exchange theory as their tool for investigating intergenerational relationships. In Izuhara's edited volume *Ageing and Intergenerational Relations: Family Reciprocity from a Global Perspective* (2010), numerous contributors theorised intergenerational relationship research. Phillipson (2010) explained social exchange theory by stating that eldercare is seen as a reward for having undertaken parenthood responsibilities. The exchanges involved in this labour of service include economic and emotional support. Social exchange theory originated from the concept of economic exchange, based on binary oppositional perspectives of 'give-take', 'cost-payment', and 'reward-punishment', as identified by Huang (2011). Even though social exchange theory is concerned with social morality, emotional support, and exchange of resources in terms of both generations' social relations and interactions, it is highly influenced by economic exchange, as also noted by Huang (2011). It easily ignores the social and cultural attributes of intergenerational relationships, such as love, emotional support, and social obligations (Huang, 2011).

To overcome social exchange theory's utilitarianist bias, Ganong and Coleman (2014) and Liou (2011) adopted reciprocity theory into research on intergenerational relationships. They identified that resource, time, and emotional exchange are mutual to both generations. This is not just a simple contractual relationship, according to Ganong and Coleman (2014). Additionally, adult children's care for elderly parents is often influenced by certain cultural regulations (Liou, 2011); as noted by Xu (2012), in China filial piety has a profound influence on intergenerational interactions, and this cultural value is reinforced through communication and exchange between parents and children.

In contemporary global research on intergenerational relationships, intergenerational solidarity (and conflict) theory feature prominently. According to Izuhara (2010), in order to conceptualise the intergenerational relationship, multiple relevant factors should be taken into account. In addition to the exchange of knowledge and resources between generations, other factors include conflicts of interest, values, and ambivalence. Phillipson (2010) pointed out that the currently dominant intergenerational solidarity–conflict model within the research arena of intergenerational relationships recognises that the complexity of the intergenerational relationship should not be seen as something solely based on reciprocity or the equality of exchange. Izuhara (2010) also contended that intergenerational conflict, such as the current prevalent conflict between traditional collective family values and modern individualism and self-autonomy and other unilateral feelings and interests, has resulted in the ambiguity of discursive meanings. According to Izuhara (2010), current research on intergenerational relationships has mainly focused on functional dimensions, such as the financial flow between generations and caregiving behaviours. How to achieve the addition of a full range of subjective dimensions, including emotional and cognitive aspects of people's experiences, to intergenerational relationship studies has not yet been properly explored, as suggested by Guo et al. (2012). In the next section, I will examine the literature exploring filial piety through the lens of intergenerational solidarity theory.

Currently, perhaps the internationally most popular theory used in research on intergenerational relationships is intergenerational solidarity theory. Luo and Zhan (2011) used intergenerational solidarity theory to consider and analyse the connections between multiple phenomena that characterise filial piety. Their study focused on older persons' own assessment of their children's level of filial piety. In general, they found that older persons were accepting of the geographic disruptions related to modernisation, yet did not think their children were less 'pious for leaving home' (Luo & Zhan, 2011, p. 69). The older persons considered their children to be more pious the more financial support they provided.

Intergenerational solidarity theory evaluates intergenerational solidarity in terms of the levels of 'associational, affectual, consensual, functional, normative, and structural' components in the relationship (Bengtson & Robert, 1991, p. 857). Some of these components are especially interesting and helpful in constructing a Foucauldian discourse analysis and establishing its orienting questions. For example, Luo and Zhan (2011) pointed out that care should be used in distinguishing between filial piety as a personal trait and as a more general social phenomenon or norm, 'with appreciation for the variability of individual manifestations and the way these are negotiated in particular cases between parent and child' (p. 71). According to Luo and Zhan (2011), personal expressions of filial piety are also modified as state services extend the definition of the forms of care due to older persons into the social and policy sphere, and partly diffuse the obligations of filial piety among a wider and increasingly accepted set of actors beyond only children.

Transactional/reciprocal elements are also entering into filial piety discourse, as urban housing challenges, for example, faced by migrant peasant workers. Young migrant peasant workers may also separate from their own children, as well as their elders, when they migrate (Luo & Zhan, 2011). They may then depend on their own parents for childcare in exchange, explicitly or otherwise, for remittances of financial support (Luo & Zhan, 2011). All these factors, identified through the lens of intergenerational solidarity theory, can contribute to a discursive analysis of filial piety.

Current research using intergenerational solidarity theory on issues around filial piety has a tendency to overvalue quantitative data and neglect qualitative data. Reconsidered from the perspective of broader academic trends, the article by Luo and Zhan (2011) discussed above describes intergenerational solidarity theory fundamentally as correlating 'functional solidarity' (i.e., forms and sources of intergenerational support) with normative solidarity (i.e., direct expressions of filial piety). In other words, this theoretical perspective points to a programme of direct empirical analysis of paired variables. I believe that intergenerational solidarity theory is a rich tool for filling in a detailed empirical picture of phenomena associated with filial piety, but that this analysis has serious limitations. It can in fact become a sort of empirical 'lucky dip' of phenomena if it fails to serve as a context for a more engaged and subjective discourse analysis. For example, a review of articles citing intergenerational solidarity theory highlights the kind of empirical questions such work tends to address. Zimmer and Kwong (2003) asked whether larger or smaller families provide more support to an aged parent. Zhan et al. (2008) asked whether children are still perceived as pious after placing their elderly parents in institutions. Xie and Zhu (2009) asked whether sons or daughters contribute more money to their parents. Giles and Mu (2007) asked whether the poor health of parents makes their children less likely to migrate. These questions are perhaps useful to enable one big aspect of the topic to be pinned down, yet fail to shed light on the hidden reasoning and mechanisms. They are useful in providing contextual information for my research, yet perhaps border on the edge of over-objectifying research subjects.

Another objection to, or perhaps limitation of, intergenerational solidarity theory relates to the usefulness of simplified quantitative modelling itself. At the most extreme level, sociological literature following this model tends to lead towards conclusions that assign a binary value to filial piety as a positive or negative thing. If it is a positive thing, the researcher then goes on to see whether some other variable is associated with generating more or less filial piety. It is the purpose of discourse analysis to instead consider the complexity of a subject and its discursive formation. If we are talking about subjective concepts like filial piety, then to some extent qualitative methodology and discourse analysis may lead to more compelling findings than the accumulation of quantitatively measurable variables.

Intergenerational solidarity theory seems to have an important role to play in building up research questions, points of reference, and empirical data that can be brought to a discourse analysis, but the discourse analysis itself takes the questions to a more compelling level. While it is important not to denigrate any formal project aimed at empirically validating a scientific hypothesis, in some cases such a discursive subjective demonstration merely adds to simple, empirical, and direct testimony. At some point it seems more important, and more sociologically relevant, to understand the complex manifestations of filial piety in more directly intuitive terms, to empathetically understand the terms of a particular negotiation or discourse among a particular group of people.

Discourse Analysis and Filial Piety

My research is fundamentally grounded in Foucauldian discourse analysis, and such an analysis requires an extensive review of the contexts for, as well as the contents of, the discourse of filial piety itself. For example, Lin (2013) placed a particular emphasis on understanding gender distinctions in the discourse about filial piety. His analysis is focused on 'highlight[ing] the under-researched notion of internal migrant men as a gendered category' (p. 105). He came to understand this as an unexpectedly complex inquiry. In particular, his work captures an evolving element of reflexivity and relationality in the way migrant men, within the social networks they interact with within 'the family and the workplace', come to define a series of issues relating to their own 'self-representation' and 'identity formation' (Lin, 2013, p. 105).

My research draws on Lin's (2013) notion of a relational self in an angle of complexity of the discursive formation of the self, instead of predominantly on identity formation. Lin (2013) identifies feminist discourse analysis as 'producing a more dynamic embodiment… of the self' (p. 109). Drawing on the Chinese notion of a relational self, such analysis directs attention not only to the multiple contexts of self-formation but to the continually evolving nature of the filial self. It involves the individual in a continuing dialogue with 'cultural norms' and 'behavioural expectations', but Lin noted, it 'never restrains creativity and possibility in different social contexts' (Lin, 2013, p. 109).

Lin (2013) took a theoretical interest in looking at discourse through power relations and by considering how power is exercised. In specific connection with filial piety, my research draws in part on Lin's engagement with self-formation and applies it more broadly in a family and kinship context, using a Foucauldian discourse analysis as a dynamic way of considering the fundamental power issues in question. Lin (2013) described and explicated the dialogue and power relations between (i.e., the discursive relations among) cultural expectations, individual improvisations, and engagement with the politically actionable social, economic, and political consequences of modernisation in China as related specifically to filial piety. The interactions and power relations between these elements help my research, in Lin's terms, to answer the questions of 'what enables their positioning in social actions and the meaning and the construction of their relational role and self-identity' (Lin, 2013, p. 110).

Apart from scholars such as Lin, there are also other scholars who have taken an interest in the discursive analysis of filial piety. Edward R. Canda (2013) focused on the evolution and transformation of Confucian ideals under 'contemporary social conditions' (p. 213). Canda noted that 'within social work and gerontology scholarship… filial piety is [currently] contested as being a positive or negative influence on family life and social welfare policy' (p. 213). And yet, in a great deal of discourse, the concept of filial piety tends to be reified, oversimplified, and treated as an unproblematic concept, except in a crude evaluation of its positive or negative effects (Canda, 2013). It is important to engage with the full complexity and potential flexibility of the concept of filial piety, as well as with its possibilities for dynamic transformation, in order to describe how it fits into discourses relating to China's modernisation.

Some research that has employed discourse analysis has more directly confronted the need to develop a conceptual vocabulary and a methodology of study that capture the fluidity, subjectivity, and contested nature of filial piety. For example, Liu (2008) looked closely at how 22 Chinese young adults negotiated their identity as filial selves in interactions with their parents. The article is helpful in clarifying the diverse ways that the notion of filial piety became embedded in direct parent–child relationship discourses. Moreover, while the investigation suggested a set of issues that can be associated with filial piety, it avoided any strict definition of the concept and aimed to sensitise the reader to the flexible, evolving, and negotiated nature of the term, which is better envisioned as a field of discourse rather than a fixed objective reality.

From what was discussed earlier in this chapter about the strong sociological focus on quantitative data in existing literature, it may be even more urgent for researchers to do more careful, discourse-oriented work to capture the way Chinese people themselves think and talk about questions addressed by academic sociologists, and such work should lead to findings that are flexible, receptive to the different positions taken by different participants in the discourse, and open to evolution over time.

A Theoretical and Methodological Debate Between Western and Chinese Approaches to Research

A broad issue in the sociological literature on filial piety is the question of western methodology versus Chinese research-related considerations. Current literature on filial piety has either fully adopted western methodology or has failed to develop a comprehensive Chinese methodology. To compensate for the lack of Chinese research tools for exploring contemporary filial discourse, some scholars have emphasised the moral persuasion of a Confucian model rather than remaining open-minded about how filial piety is experienced by Chinese people today. In the wake of the Chinese government's promotion of filial piety within the last decade in order to build harmonious familial relationships and enhance social order, Guo (2011) pointed out that the ancient Confucian morality system incorporated a need to ensure provisional care for parents, founded on ethical and emotional bonding between parents and children. This system drew strength from social and political forces and was very successful; today's China could also learn from such a Confucian morality system being integrated into families, schools, and society. Yao (2007) reckoned that the ancient Confucian discourse of filial piety contained an essence that could help to not only facilitate the construction of family morality but also build a more general sense of social responsibility. Scholars such as Xiao (2005), Tang (2006), and Li (2007) discussed the importance of promoting filial education in schools, including universities, because filial culture and perception were absent in those spaces in current Chinese society. The above-mentioned research tends to identify a decline in filial perception and then prescribe a solution that is borrowed from ancient times and discuss the social functions of such solutions. This approach excludes analysis of current social contexts and ignores people's subjective constructions of relevant concepts and behaviours; a simple borrowing from ancient ways may not be as effective as one might think, since the social context has changed.

On the other hand, some Chinese scholars fully adopt western research tools on issues involving filial piety and care. According to Zhou et al. (2016), some Chinese researchers saw filial piety itself as a cultural resource for strengthening intergenerational solidarity and ensuring elder-care in contemporary Chinese society. For example, Meng's (2006) case study, undertaken in Sichuan province, demonstrated that Confucian filial piety has a positive influence on facilitating intergenerational solidarity.

The underlying question is whether the conceptual categories in western academic literature are really applicable to Chinese experience or are truly useful in the analysis of Chinese cases, or whether more localised methodologies should be developed to reflect Chinese social reality. The issue perhaps can be addressed more subtly in discourse terms: can the methods used in western academic discourse analysis really help to illuminate the way filial piety is actually manifested and thought and talked about in China? To answer this, we need to first look at the history of sociology in China.

The History of Sociology in China: Underdevelopment of Localised Sociology

The issue of culturally alien categories in Chinese sociology is often discussed through the filter of tension between western Enlightenment and Chinese Confucian (and other philosophical) values. Wen and Chen (2013) suggested that at the beginning of the twentieth century, a 'strong cultural enlightenment movement' (the New Culture Movement) developed in China that was heavily based on imported western values (p. 200). It represented a comprehensive critique of traditional Chinese values and institutions that were held to reflect backwardness and barriers to modernisation by certain Chinese elites. These western or modern values included 'democracy and the primacy of science' (Wen & Chen, 2013, p. 201).

Chinese sociology was underdeveloped in terms of 'localising' the discipline, and tended to be *objectified* (lacking an interest in qualitative research), in particular during the last century before economic reform (Ma, 1998). The western and quantitatively focused orientation of the discipline may be traced, according to Ma (1998), to the existence of over 144 academic positions in sociology in Chinese universities, more than two-thirds of them occupied by quantitative scholars trained in the United States or Europe in the early twentieth century. Chinese academic sociology, according to Ma (1998), focused on issues considered crucial to China's modernisation and development, including 'social stratification, rural economy, population, urban living costs, labor, etc.' (p. 46). Therefore, there has been a lack of qualitative research and qualitative data from the beginning of sociology in China, and also a lack of development of a unique Chinese sociology. After 1949, sociology as a discipline was deprecated as a 'capitalist pseudoscience' and suppressed until the reform era began in 1979 (Ma, 1998, p. 46). Especially during the Cultural Revolution, the development of sociology was almost fully constrained.

Development of 'Localising' Sociological Theories and Methodologies in Recent Years

The new enlightenment movement mentioned above in turn tended to generate a Confucian reaction, especially in recent years. Wen and Chen (2013) maintained that distinctive elements of Chinese culture, including Confucian culture, have the power to shape Chinese society and history in distinct ways that make western sociological categories only imperfectly relevant to the analysis of Chinese phenomena. Tu (2000) expressed faith in Confucian values and their role in shaping modern Chinese society, arguing that the 'high expectations of Confucian scholars throughout Chinese history' naturally result in an 'expansive expectation that Confucian ideas can dramatically change reality' (Tu, 2000, p. 200). While sympathising with Chinese cultural resentment about the erosive effect of western thinking on valued traditions, Tu's (2000) argument needs to be considered critically, especially when the researcher adopts the methodological tool of discourse analysis to investigate a matter with strong Chinese and Confucian elements.

Recently, it has become better recognised that sociology needs to be adapted to the unique Chinese context. Bian (2002), in his review of Chinese academic sociology since the 1980s, suggested that the re-established discipline has displayed a tension between a desire to reintegrate with global academic norms in the post-Maoist era and a 'persistent search for a rooting in Chinese society' (p. 139). Bian (2002) suggested that from the west, and especially from American academic sociology, Chinese sociology has acquired a relatively new emphasis on 'standard survey methods to collect systematic data and form theoretical and substantive analyses about such issues as institutional change, changing patterns of social stratification, mechanisms of social mobility, and the centrality of social networks in social life' (p. 139). More recently, however, a 2015 international academic conference entitled *Doing Post-Western Sociology* (cited in Roulleau-Berger, 2016) attempted to consolidate an agenda reflecting innovative far-reaching trends, notably those led by French and Chinese sociology. Trends that were noted included an emerging emphasis on questions of 'domination, agency and subjectivation', as well as issues and processes involving 'individuation, modernities, and experiences', and the reinterpretation of 'institutions, norms, and resistance' (Roulleau-Berger, 2016). These issues place emerging trends in Chinese sociology at the forefront of attempts to overcome more traditional quantitative and reifying approaches to sociological inquiry. According to Sun (2002), Chinese sociology has to develop localised methodologies for Chinese social matters.

Internationally, sinology (an academic field specialising in China, cross-cultural knowledge production, and Chinese-western studies) has developed over a long time, since the missionaries first wrote about China in the thirteenth century (Chen, 2014). In the early nineteenth century, sinology became an official research school in Europe and its centre transferred to North America in the twentieth century; it was heavily influenced by Orientalism since its start (Fokkema, 2011; Miller, 1996). Said criticised Orientalism for containing a strong sentiment of western centralism and political hegemony (Said, 2003). Orientalism consists of two elements: (1) the differences of epistemology and methodology between the east and the west cannot be solved; (2) due to the dominance of western discursive hegemony, the relationship between the east and the west presents the relationship between the dominant and the dominated. Since World War II, the research focus of sinology has shifted from ancient Chinese civilisation to current problems in China (Chen, 2014). The most recent transformation in sinology began at the turn of the twenty-first century and is still in progress. Its main purpose is to integrate Chinese and western perspectives, creating new opportunities for Chinese and western academic circles as a comprehensive research field (Chen, 2009).

The concept of sinologism, first proposed by scholars in China and internationally, refers to one important aspect of the discursive or ideological nature of sinological studies. Inspired by Said's critique of Orientalism, sinologism expresses a conscious criticism of cultural hegemony in knowledge production (N. Zhou, 2018). Gu and Zhou (2018) believed that the growing interest in sinology in the Chinese academic community is related to the cultural consciousness in the process of China's rise, which involves the criticism of western sinology on its misinterpretation and misunderstanding of China. This kind of misinterpretation and misunderstanding belongs to a type of discourse of subjective choice, construction, and presentation. It is subject to the system of western cultural hegemony (Barmé, 2005).

In China's local intellectual circles, sinologistic influence is also very common. On the one hand, self-colonisation of the sinologistic mentality is prevalent. Even some well-known scholars worship western sinology and regard it as an academic norm (X. Zhou, 2018). Yang (2016) pointed out that for more than a century, Chinese traditional culture and knowledge have been gradually dominated and excluded by the western hegemonic discourse, so that Chinese knowledge has become a kind of 'academic data', as texts that can be analysed in research. On the other hand, X. Zhou (2018, p. 77) pointed out another bias in Chinese academic circles, i.e., civilisation supremacy, i.e., that 'one tends to believe in the supremacy of one's own civilisation or culture'. This tendency often hinders Chinese scholars' recognition of the advantages of western social science theories and methods or of the valid views of western scholars. The common prejudices and misunderstandings in both Chinese and international academic circles rely on how one views and deals with the other's culture. Many Chinese scholars with this bias seek their entire inspiration from China's historical and cultural traditions and totally reject western theories (Tang & Hou, 2003; Wang, 2011). They often use the limited philosophical concepts in ancient Chinese literature to explain current social phenomena, but lack in critical analysis, so they cannot form advanced theories or methodological innovation. This ignores not only the comprehensiveness of Chinese traditional philosophy but also the complexity of modernity and Chineseness in the contemporary Chinese context, as well as the historical origin of sociology, which was in the west. Therefore, sinologism has become an important issue in the development of the theory and methodology of cultural integration of sinology.

N. Zhou (2018) claims that progress in solving sinological problems depends on how to avoid using pre-existing views and prejudices to examine other cultures and civilisations. In my opinion, this raises a more complicated problem more Chinese sociologists, because we have to examine our own culture from at least some perspectives of western theory and methodology, as sociology not only originated in the west but is still dominated by western theories and methods globally. According to N. Zhou, to understand other needs, we should first seek common ground, which will create an effective possibility for entering into a process of equal dialogue. Standaert (2015) also believes that the solution for sinologism is essentially about an art of *inbetweenness*, which strives to find a common ground through which cross-cultural understanding can be carried out (see also White, 1991; Watsuji, 2011).

One increasingly popular way of operationalising the notion of 'Chinese sociology', but perhaps not the most useful way, is by a refinement of terminology. For instance, in his book *Reconstructing the Confucian Dao*, Adler (2014) claimed that Confucianism in Chinese does not mean Confucius and -ism but rather *ru xue* 儒学 (scholarly learning/knowledge). *Ru xue* is comprised of the teachings not only of Confucius but also of his followers and other scholars with similar theoretical underpinnings. A refined and localised terminology might speak for itself without long-winded theorisation. Liang and Luo (2012), for example, proposed that more western-type considerations of *successful ageing* or *active ageing* (emphasising individual needs) be replaced by what they see as the more Chinese concept of *harmonious ageing* (focusing on the interdependent nature of family, friends, and social relationships of elders). Such a conceptual renovation, the authors suggested, can help 'ease the tension between activity and disengagement theories' and can 'emphasize the interdependent nature of human beings' (Liang & Luo, 2012, p. 327). Such a discourse, the authors believed, can inform and benefit both academic work and policy initiatives, by 'improving the cross-cultural relevance of associated investigations' (p. 327).

Such a refinement of terminology reflects an attempt to integrate the similarities and differences. The point in successfully localising western methodology into the Chinese context is not the differences between the west and China but how the differences are dealt with. More importantly, the similarities between the two cultures and theoretical traditions need to be realised first to establish a channel for equal dialogue and mutual communication.

Conclusion

This chapter reviewed recent literature on adult children's care towards their parents, filial piety, and discourses of filial piety in contemporary Chinese society. The review first introduced literature that showed a relationship between informal family care for aged parents and filial piety. I identified a claim commonly made in the literature that there has been a decline in filial practices and perceptions in rural China in the post-economic reform era, in terms of adult children's informal caregiving for parents in need. In that literature, this perceived decline of filial piety is related to contextual changes in contemporary Chinese society. Neoliberalism has often been blamed as the culprit. Researchers have seldom investigated the subjective care experiences of adult children, in particular migrant peasant workers, and their construction of the filial self, and this is reflected in a lack of literature on this topic.

The second part of the chapter considered the general and broad theoretical points of view on filial piety reflected in the literature. Several theories that frequently emerge in the literature were discussed and critiqued to reveal the theoretical gap my research addresses. Modernisation theory treats the decline in filial piety as an inevitable outcome of a 'western' path towards modernisation. Intergenerational solidarity theory takes a quantitative position in investigating filial discourse. Research that uses discourse analysis provides a way of looking at filial piety to potentially arrive at refreshing insights, challenging current mainstream research methodologies and theoretical tools. A research focus among Chinese scholars on Confucian discourse around filial piety revealed a gap in western methodologies leading to a failure to examine the highly cultural Chinese context of filial piety.

In the final section, a review of the history of sociology in China begins to identify the lack of appropriate localised methodologies, something that is also evident in sinological studies. The solution lies in how common ground between western methodologies and Chinese culture can be reached and how differences might be dealt with. In the next two chapters, I provide a more detailed explanation of the specific theoretical and methodological approach of my research, including a more thorough justification for the combining of Foucauldian theory and Chinese philosophies (mainly Confucianism). I examine differences between Chinese and western philosophies, and more importantly similarities between Chinese philosophies and Foucault's theories. I explain how I drew from similarities between Chinese philosophies, especially Confucianism, and Foucault's theories to identify a localised Foucauldian discourse analysis tool for my research.

References

Adler, J. A. (2014). *Reconstructing the Confucian dao*. State University of New York Press.

Alasuutari, P. (1995). *Researching culture: Qualitative method and cultural studies*. Sage.

Barmé, G. R. (2005). Towards a new Sinology. *Chinese Studies Association of Australia Newsletter, 31*(May), 4–9.

Bengtson, V. L., & Robert, E. L. R. (1991). Intergenerational solidarity in aging families: An example of formal theory construction. *Journal of Marriage and Family, 53*(4), 856–70. https://onlinelibrary.wiley.com/journal/17413737

Bian, Y. (2002). Sociological research on reform-era China. *Issues & Studies, 38–39*(4–1), 139–174. http://issues.nccu.edu.tw/

Canda, E. R. (2013). Filial piety and care for elders: A contested Confucian virtue reexamined. *Journal of Ethnic and Cultural Diversity in Social Work, 22*(3–4), 213–234. https://doi.org/10.1080/15313204.2013.843134

Chen, J. (2014). Earl miner: New sinology through comparative literature. *Neohelicon, 41*, 427–443. https://doi.org/10.1007/s11059-014-0259-4

Chen, L. L. (2009). Review: sinographies: Writing China. In E. Hayot, H. Saussy, & S. G. Yao (Eds.), *The China Journal, 62,* 149–151.

Chen, R., & Hu, Q. (2015). Research on the function of family care and support systems under the trend toward social aged care 社会化养老趋势下家庭照料的作用及支持体系研究. *City Observation 城市观察, 3,* 126–31. http://csgc.xueshu.com/

Cheung, C. K., & Kwan, A.Y.-H. (2009). The erosion of filial piety by modernisation in Chinese cities. *Ageing & Society, 29*(2), 179–198. https://doi.org/10.1017/S0144686X08007836

Ding, C. (2003). *The historical construction of traditional filial piety and its reconstruction in contemporary Chinese society 传统"孝道"的历史建构及其在当代的重建.* Yunnan Normal University 云南师范大学.

Fan, R. (2007). Which care? Whose responsibility? And why family? A Confucian account of long-term care for the elderly. *Journal of Medicine and Philosophy, 32*(5), 495–517. https://doi.org/10.1080/03605310701626331

Fokkema, D. (2011). *Perfect worlds: Utopian fiction in China and the West.* Amsterdam University Press.

Ganong, L., & Coleman, M. (2014). Qualitative research on family relationships. *Journal of Social and Personal Relationships, 31*(4), 451–459. https://doi.org/10.1177/0265407514520828

Giles, J., & Mu, R. (2007). Elderly parent health and the migration decisions of adult children: Evidence from rural China. *Demography, 44*(2), 265–288. https://doi.org/10.1353/dem.2007.0010

Gruijters, R. J. (2017). Family care-giving and living arrangements of functionally impaired elders in rural China. *Ageing and Society, 37*(3), 633–647. https://doi.org/10.1017/S0144686X15001397

Gu, M. D., & Zhou, X. (2018). Sinology, sinologism, and new sinology. *Contemporary Chinese Thought, 49*(1), 1–6, https://doi.org/10.1080/10971467.2018.1534494

Guo, K. (2011). Inspiration of traditional filial education for modern morality/ethical education 传统孝道教育特点及对现代德育的启示. *Hunan Technology College Publication 湖南科技学院学报, 32*(2), 63–65. http://fabiao.xmqikan.com/index.html

Guo, M., Chi, I., & Silverstein, M. (2012). The structure of intergenerational relations in rural China: A latent class analysis. *Journal of Marriage and Family, 74*(5), 1114–1128. https://doi.org/10.1111/j.1741-3737.2012.01014.x

Ho, D. Y. F. (1994). Filial piety, authoritarian moralism, and cognitive conservatism in Chinese societies. *Genetic, Social, and General Psychology Monographs, 120*(3), 349–365. https://www.ncbi.nlm.nih.gov

Hooyman, N. R., & Kiyak, H. A. (2008). Opportunities and challenges of informal caregiving. In N. R. Hooyman & H. A. Kiyak (Eds.), *Social gerontology: A multidisciplinary perspective* (pp. 385–428). Allyn & Bacon.

Huang, J. (2011). *The reproduction of filial piety in a community: Discourse and practice*. Social Sciences Academic Press.

Huang, Y. (2006). *Investigation of motivation of adult children for caring for aged parents* 成年子女对老年父母的照顾动机探析. Doctoral dissertation, Huazhong Normal University, Wuhan. http://shxy.ccnu.edu.cn

Ikels, C. (2004). *Filial piety: Practice and discourse in contemporary East Asia*. Stanford University Press.

Ikels, C. (2006). Economic reform and intergenerational relationships in China. *Oxford Development Studies, 34*(4), 387–400. https://doi.org/10.1080/13600810601045619

Izuhara, M. (Ed.). (2010). *Ageing and intergenerational relations: Family reciprocity from a global perspective*. Policy.

Ji, Q. (2009). Literature review of filial culture of mainland China in the last ten years 近十年中国大陆孝文化研究综述. *Social Science Commentary 社会科学评论* (3), 123–130. http://www.cssn.cn/xspj/

Jones, S. (1985). The analysis of depth interviews. In R. Walker (Ed.), *Applied qualitative research* (pp. 56–70). Gower.

Kuo, T., & Tsou, H. (2016). Filial piety and caregiver burden among Taiwanese family caregivers of older parents in institutions (Abstract for presentation given at the GSA 2016 Annual Scientific Meeting). *The Gerontologist, 56*(Suppl_3), 505. https://doi.org/10.1093/geront/gnw162.2038

Lai, D. W. (2010). Filial piety, caregiving appraisal, and caregiving burden. *Research on Aging, 32*(2), 200–223. https://doi.org/10.1177/0164027509351475

Lee, A. E. Y. (1997). *Family social support patterns of the Chinese elderly in Beijing, Shanghai, Guangzhou and Los Angeles: The role of filial piety*. University of California Press.

Li, H. (2007). Meaning and practice of filial culture in university culture-building 论孝文化在高校校园文化建设中的意义与实践. *Exam Weekly 考试周刊2*(2). http://www.58zazhi.com/

Li, H., Wang, M., Huang, H., & Zhao, H. (2009). Investigation of care burden for elders with chronic conditions对老年慢性病患者照顾者家庭负担的调查分析. *China Nursing Magazine中华护理杂志, 44*(6), 561–564. http://zh.zhhlzzs.com/CN/0254-1769/home.shtml

Li, X., & Zhao, H. (2009). Literature review on family caregivers and their ability to care老年人家庭照顾者及其照顾能力研究现状. *China Care Magazine 中华护理杂志* (11), 1051–1053. http://zh.zhhlzzs.com/CN/0254-1769/home.shtml

Liang, J., & Luo, B. (2012). Towards a discourse shift in social gerontology: From successful aging to harmonious aging. *Journal of Aging Studies, 26*(3), 327–334. https://doi.org/10.1016/j.jaging.2012.03.001

Lin, X. (2013). *Gender, modernity and male migrant workers in China: Becoming a 'modern' man*. Routledge.

Liu, F. (2008). Negotiating the filial self: Young-adult only-children and intergenerational relationships in China. *Young, 16*(4), 409–430. https://doi.org/10.1177/110330880801600404

Liu, N., & Yu, X. (2008). Construction of a long-term care system for elders through filial tradition 论我国孝道传统下老年人长期照护制度的构建. *Southwest University (Social Science) 西南大学学报(社会科学版), 34*(5), 106–110. http://xbbjb.swu.edu.cn/

Liu, W. (2012). The diminishing of filial piety? The perception, behaviour, and relevant affecting factors of adult children caring for aged parents孝道衰落? 成年子女支持父母的观念, 行为及其影响因素. *Youth Research 青年研究, 2*, 22–32. http://www.zhazhi.com/qikan/shxzx/shx/1355.html

Liou, C. L. (2011). Review: Ageing and intergenerational relations: Family reciprocity from a global perspective by Misa Izuhara. *Journal of Intergenerational Relationships, 9*(1), 98–102. https://doi.org/10.1080/15350770.2011.544219

Lu, J. (2016). *Rural elders' filial perception and evaluation of children's filial behaviour 当代农村老年人的孝道观念与对子女孝行为评价研究*. Doctoral dissertation, Huazhong Agricultural University, Wuhan.

Lum, Y. S. T., Yan, C. W. E., Ho, H. Y. A., Shum, H. Y. M., Wong, H. Y. G., Lau, M. M. Y., & Wang, J. F. (2016). Measuring filial piety in the 21st century: Development, factor structure, and reliability of the 10-item Contemporary Filial Piety Scale. *Journal of Applied Gerontology, 35*(11), 1235–1247. https://doi.org/10.1177/0733464815570664

Luo, C. (2003). *Selected writings on Chinese ancient filial piety 中国古代孝道资料选编*. Shandong University Publisher 山东大学出版社.

Luo, B., & Zhan, H. (2011). Filial piety and functional support: Understanding intergenerational solidarity among families with migrated children in rural China. *Ageing International, 37*(1), 69–92. https://doi.org/10.1007/s12126-011-9132-1

Ma, R. (1998). Institutionalization of sociology in China. In S.-H. Lee (Ed.), *Heritage, challenges, perspectives: Sociology in East Asia and its struggle for creativity* (pp. 45–49). International Sociological Association.

Meng, C. (2006). Filial culture facilitates intergenerational solidarity: An example from Sichuan province 孝文化促进代际和谐——以四川省为例. *Southwestern Ethnic University Publishing (Social Science)西南民族大学学报(人文社科版), 27*(11), 53–56. http://xnmzxbsk.ijournal.cn/ch/index.aspx

Miller, F. R. (1996). Review: Communist China in retrospect: East European Sinologists remember the first fifteen years of the PRC by Marie-Luise Nath. *The China Journal, 35,* 187–189. https://doi.org./https://doi.org/10.2307/2950308

Pan, J., Zhong, J., & Zhou, H. (2006). Study of filial culture and rural non-material 'civilisation/culture' 孝文化与农村精神文明的调查研究. *Literature and History Encyclopedia文史博览* (4), 59–61. http://wenshibolan.com/

Phillipson, C. (2010). Globalisation, global ageing and intergenerational change. In M. Izuhara (Ed.), *Ageing and intergenerational relations: Family reciprocity from a global perspective* (pp. 13–28). Policy.

Pope, C., Ziebland, S., & Mays, N. (2000). Qualitative research in health care: Analysing qualitative data. *British Medical Journal, 320*(7227), 114–116. https://doi.org/10.1136/bmj.320.7227.114

Punch, K. (2005). *Introduction to social research: Quantitative and qualitative approaches* (2nd ed.). SAGE.

Roulleau-Berger, L. (2016). *Post-Western revolution in sociology: From China to Europe*. Brill.

Said, E. W. (2003). *Orientalism*. Penguin.

Standaert, N. (2015). Don't mind the gap: Sinology as an art of in-betweenness. *Philosophy Compass, 10*(2), 91–103. https://doi.org/10.1111/phc3.12199

Sun, L. (2002). A sociology towards practice 迈向实践的社会学. *Jianghai Study 江海学刊* (3), 84–90. http://www.jhxk.cn/CN/volumn/home.shtml

Tang, J., & Hou, J. (2003). Indigenisation possibilities for social science research 试论社会科学研究的本土化进路. *Tianjing Social Science 天津社会科学, 3*, 39–42.

Tang, M. (2006). A discussion of the contemporary meaning of traditional filial culture: From adolescent education and elder care and respect 浅论传统孝文化的时代意义——从青少年教育和养老敬老谈起. *Qinghai Social Science 青海社会科学* (1), 20–22. http://www.qhass.org/

Tu, W. (2000). Implications of the rise of 'Confucian' East Asia. *Daedalus, 129*(1), 195–218. https://www.amacad.org/content/publications/publicationListing.aspx?i=135

Wang, S. (2011). Localisation of sociology from the 1980s in China 20世纪80年代以来中国社会科学本土化研究的问题与展望. *Inner Mongolia Ethnic University Journal (Social Science) 内蒙古民族大学学报(社会科学版) 17*(3): 98–100.

Wang, Y. (2014). *Chinese traditional filial piety and contemporary rural family elder care research 中国传统孝道思想与当代农村家庭养老研究*. QingHai Normal University 青海师范大学.

Watsuji, T. (2011). *Fûdo, le milieu humain*. Trans. Augustin Berque. CNRS.

Wei, H., & Zhong, Z. (2016). Pragmatic analysis of adult children's parental care: Intergenerational exchange, filial culture and structural constraints 代际交换、孝道文化与结构制约:子女赡养行为的实证分析. *Nanjing Agriculture University Publisher (Social Science) 南京农业大学学报(社会科学版)* (1), 144–155. http://www.cqvip.com/qk/85303X/

Wen, H., & Chen, D. (2013). 'Confucian cultural fallacy' in the 20th century Chinese enlightenment movement. *Frontiers of Philosophy in China, 8*(2), 199–214. http://hep.calis.edu.cn

Wen, X. (2017). *The reason and solution for the weakening functionality of filial piety in rural aged care 孝道在我国农村养老中功能弱化的原因及对策.* Doctoral dissertation, North University of China, Taiyuan.

White, R. (1991). *The middle ground: Indians, empires, and republics in the Great Lakes Region, 1650–1815.* Cambridge University Press.

Willig, C. (2001). *Introducing qualitative research in psychology: Adventures in theory and method.* Open University Press.

Xiao, L. D., Wang, J., He, G.-P., De Bellis, A., Verbeeck, J., & Kyriazopoulos, H. (2014). Family caregiver challenges in dementia care in Australia and China: A critical perspective. *BMC Geriatrics, 14*(1), 6–6. https://doi.org/10.1186/1471-2318-14-6

Xiao, Q. (2000). Traditional filial piety and contemporary elder care传统孝道与当代养老模式. *Northwestern University Publication (Social Science) 西北师大学报:社会科学版* (2), 101–105. http://mall.cnki.net/magazine/magadetail/XBSD201502.htm

Xiao, Q. (2005). Confucian filial piety and contemporary Chinese ethical education 儒家孝道与当代中国伦理教育. *Nanchang University Publication (Social Science) 南昌大学学报(人文社会科学版), 36*(1), 1–6. http://qks.ncu.edu.cn/CN/model/index.shtml

Xie, Y., & Zhu, H. (2009). Do sons or daughters give more money to parents in urban China? *Journal of Marriage and Family, 71*(1), 174–186. https://doi.org/10.1111/j.1741-3737.2008.00588.x

Xu, J. (2012). Filial piety and intergenerational communication in China: A nationwide study. *Journal of International Communication, 18*(1), 33–48. https://doi.org/10.1080/13216597.2012.662466

Yao, J. (2007). Thoughts on the value of Chinese traditional filial piety in modern ethics and morality construction 中国传统孝道在现代道德建设中的价值思考. *Anyang Normal College Press安阳师范学院学报, 6*, 35–36.

Yang, Y. (2016). The ups and downs of contemporary *guoxue* 近现代国学之跌宕起伏. *New West: Mid Theory 新西部: 中旬·理论* (8), 97–98. http://www.cnki.com.cn/Journal/J-J1-XXBL.htm

Zeng, Z. (2002). Confucian filial piety's emergence and variation 儒家孝论的发生及其变异. *Literature, History and Philosophy* 文史哲 (06), 47–53. http://www.lhp.sdu.edu.cn/

Zhan, H. J., Feng, X., & Luo, B. (2008). Placing elderly parents in institutions in urban China: A reinterpretation of filial piety. *Research on Aging, 30*(5), 543–571. https://doi.org/10.1177/0164027508319471

Zhang, J. (2000). The formation and evolution of Confucian filial piety 儒家孝道观的形成与演变. *History of Chinese Philosophy* 中国哲学史 (03), 74–79. http://www.zhazhi.com/qikan/shxzx/zzl/3484.html

Zhao, Q. (2017). Issues and relevant solutions in modern rural filial piety issues 现代农村家庭孝道中存在的问题与对策研究. *New West: Theory* 新西部:理论版 (14), 12–12. http://www.htqkw.com/article/737.html

Zhao, Z. (2017). Research review of filial culture since economic reform 改革开放以来孝文化研究述评. *Xihua University Scholarly (Philosophy and Social Science)* 西华大学学报 (哲学社会科学版), *5*, 003. http://qk.xhu.edu.cn/1908/list.htm

Zhong, X., & He, S. (2014). Negotiating intimate relationships: Family relationship and filial piety expectations of parents of only children 协商式亲密关系: 独生子女父母对家庭关系和孝道的期待. *Open Times* 开放时代, *1*(008), 155–175. http://www.opentimes.cn/

Zhou, N. (2018). "Sinologism": Rethinking the legitimacy of Sinology as knowledge. *Contemporary Chinese Thought, 49*(1), 7–12. https://doi.org/10.1080/10971467.2018.1534495

Zhou, S., Zhang, L., & Lan, X. (2016). Research review of filial culture in recent years 近年来孝道文化研究综述. *Changjiang congkang* 长江丛刊 (17), 36–37. http://128.qikan.qwfbw.com/

Zhou, X. (2018). The problems of Sinologism and strategies to cope with them. *Contemporary Chinese Thought, 49*(1), 71–80. https://doi.org/10.1080/10971467.2018.1534504

Zhu, L., Xin, R. & Gao, Q. (2019). Difficulties of returned migrant peasant workers due to work-related injuries from a realistic perspective. "可行能力"视角下因工伤残返乡农民工生存困境研究. *Jinan University Press (Social Science Edition)* 济南大学学报:社会科学版, *29*(03), 115–124. https://doi.org/10.3969/j.issn.1671-3842.2019.03.013

Zhu, M., & Liang, Y. (2006). Filial culture is the realistic choice in contemporary rural China弘扬孝文化是新农村建设的现实选择. *Guangdong Administration College Publication* 广东行政学院学报, *18*(05), 94–95. http://gdxz.Chinajournal.net.cn/WKE/WebPublication/index.aspx?mid=GDXZ

Zimmer, Z., & Kwong, J. (2003). Family size and support of older adults in urban and rural China: Current effects and future implications. *Demography, 40*(1), 23–44. https://doi.org/10.1353/dem.2003.0010

CHAPTER 4

Foucault and Chinese Traditional Philosophies (Confucianism)

Introduction

Foucault's theories are the foundation for Foucauldian discourse analysis, developed by numerous scholars over time. Important aspects of Foucault's theories that form the basis of my research's theoretical foundations will be synthesised and explained in this chapter. In the first part of this chapter, I explain these concepts and their relationship to filial piety, commencing with a discussion of what discourse means in a Foucauldian sense, and how the concept of discourse relates to power. Next follows a brief explanation of governmental discursive power and why it is of theoretical importance to include political discourse of filial piety in my research. Lastly, I discuss Foucault's conceptualisations of archaeology, genealogy, and subjectivity in relation to the discourse of filial piety.

In the second half of this chapter, three theoretical foundations that are held in common between Chinese traditional philosophies (especially Confucianism) and Foucauldian theorising are identified and explained. These theoretical commonalities are the complexity of relationality, the pragmatic nature of Chinese philosophies and Foucauldian theorising, and the importance of looking back into ancient history to understand techniques for *care of the self*. Their identification lays the groundwork for a consideration of how a Foucauldian discourse analysis can be conducted with Chineseness; the chapter builds an argument for the theoretical significance of a localised western methodology in the research arena

L. He, *Care Work, Migrant Peasant Families and Discourse of Filial Piety in China*, https://doi.org/10.1007/978-981-16-1880-2_4

of filial piety that may have broader relevance for other Chinese social matters.

Foucault's Theory in Relation to Filial Piety

Foucault's theories are significant in my own theorising on filial piety. In this section, I explain the most relevant of his theoretical ideas.

Discourse (and Power)

According to Hook (2001), in Foucauldian ideology knowledge always embodies certain discourses that follow a set of rules or regulations. Throughout Foucault's published works, from *The Archaeology of Knowledge* (1970b) to *The History of Sexuality* (1978c), he explained the mechanisms created by discourse and constructed a somewhat systematic way of historically analysing discourse. For Foucault, discourse is constructed through sets of signs/symbols, statements, and practices that are expressed and asserted as a particular way of existence (see, for example, Foucault, 1970b). Foucault did not invest in the statements themselves but rather believed that discourse goes beyond what objects and subjects symbolically represent (Foucault, 1970b). The extra 'things' discourse contains cannot be simply extracted as words or texts. Discourses enable and constrain, facilitate, and limit what can be spoken about, by whom, when, and where (Foucault,). According to Foucauldian discourse analysts such as Dreyfus and Rabinow (1982) and Smith (2008), Foucauldian scholars ask how discourse is formed and explore in what ways available discursive resources (beyond words and texts) within a particular context influence this particular discourse.

Theories on discourse can be employed to explain how social phenomena are culturally embedded. For Foucault in his early stage of theorisation, everything could be discourse. Therefore, Foucault rejected the concept of universal truth, as truth was only constructed within discourse (Foucault, 1978a). According to Dreyfus and Rabinow (1982), for Foucault, 'truth' could be narrated as nothing exists outside of discourse. In Foucault's last stage of life, he tried to engage in considerations of agency (the idea that individuals might be able to access ways of reaching a certain degree of freedom in action or thought) in relation to his explanation of care of the self.

According to Gaventa (2003), for Foucault, both agency and structure were constructed through power. Foucault claimed that power can be everywhere. It is essential to the discursive construction of knowledge and discourse, and vice versa:

> Discourses are not once and for all subservient to power or raised up against it . . . We must make allowance for the complex and unstable process whereby a discourse can be both an instrument and an effect of power, but also a hindrance, a stumbling block, a point of resistance and a starting point for an opposing strategy. Discourse transmits and produces power; it reinforces it, but also undermines and exposes it, renders it fragile and makes it possible to thwart it. (Foucault, 1978c, p. 100)

For Foucault, power was persuasive and dispersed, as opposed to possessed or owned by people or groups through coercion and manipulation (Foucault & Sheridan, 1977). 'Power is everywhere' and 'comes from everywhere', thereby it is neither a structure nor an agency (Foucault, 1998, p. 63). In my research, power is considered in relation to discourse; power relations are everywhere and come from everywhere. In keeping with Foucault's theorising, power (relations) can be productive as well as repressive and negative (Foucault, 1998). Power can both enable and constrain possibilities through discourse.

> We must cease once and for all to describe the effects of power in negative terms: it 'excludes', it 'represses', it 'censors', it 'abstracts', it 'masks', it 'conceals'. In fact power produces; it produces reality; it produces domains of objects and rituals of truth. The individual and the knowledge that may be gained of him belong to this production. (Foucault & Sheridan, 1977, p. 194)

The duality of power expressed above indicates the complexity of power relations. In the discourse of filial piety, power is exercised between individuals' various identities within family relationships. Power, just as discourse, can both constrain and enable people's sense-making.

Foucault used his dialectical conceptualising of power/knowledge to demonstrate that power is constructed through scientific understanding, acquired forms of knowledge, and truth. Foucault sees truth as produced through kinds of discourses that function to promote perceptions of what is true (Foucault, 1977a). Regular effects of power are induced by such constructed truths. In this book, concepts of what is truth and what is *natural* are overlapping (on Chinese philosophical conceptualisations of what is natural see Chapters 6 and 7). According to Edwards (2013) and Lewis (1983), there is a significant correlation between truth and naturalness in metaphysics. They contended that the ultimate truth is built on discourse of the most natural subjects and properties. For Foucault, regimes of truth are built upon scientific discourse and reinforced through scientific institutions, modern political and economic systems, education, and so on (Foucault & Sheridan, 1977). Truth is not objective but rather a set of rules and regulations that separate what is conceived to be true and false.

Discursive Formation. Foucault emphasised *discursive formation*, which in his later writings replaced his early idea of the episteme from *The Order of Things: An Archaeology of the Human Sciences* (Foucault, 1970b). The episteme refers to 'unconscious' and orderly structures that form the possibility and conditions of scientific knowledge at any given time and place (O'Farrell, 2007, p. 39). Foucault placed more importance on how and why one speaks than to specifically who speaks. Discourse is often realised in the name of 'truth' or 'knowledge' (in other words, discourse can be seen as a form of truth). The will to attain truth or knowledge propels people to practise discursiveness (Foucault, 1970b). It successfully conceals the discipline that power operates on people (Oliver, 2010). For Foucault, there is no universal or natural knowledge (Foucault, 1978a). Any knowledge is generated in the conspiracy between power and knowledge through discursive formation (May, 2006). For example, neo-Confucian discourse of filial piety was constructed through many factors, especially top-down state manipulation and other power conspiracies. Discourse is more than the ways in which meanings are represented through language, and it interacts closely with invisible constructive power. Such power constructs the world we are living in and the conceptualisation of the self. Foucault sees the self as a historical subject constructed through limited and limiting conditions; the self is produced through either the practice of power/discourse, or technologies/cultivation of the self (Foucault, 1970a).

In Foucault's early theorisation of discourse, knowledge does not come from subjective observation and life experiences but from discursive formation. For example, modern knowledge is produced through discursive formation within scientific/disciplinary discourse (Foucault, 1970b). Foucault emphasised how knowledge and power conspire with each other within certain discourses (Dreyfus & Rabinow, 1982). His concept of the episteme dictates that discursive practice cannot escape from the regulation imposed on constructs in time and place (Foucault, 1970a). The reason he stopped using the episteme was because he could not ignore the occurrence of resistance to power, which provides an opportunity for a certain freedom of agency. Both the structure side of discourse and Foucault's consideration of the agency of individuals over traditional/cultural discourse, discussed above, are in line with my research aim to investigate migrant peasant workers' sense-making of care experiences through discourses of filial piety.

Discursive Formation of Tradition and History. Foucault's theory of discourse sees the past and tradition as discursively constructed through current discourses. Hobsbawm and Ranger (1983) stated that tradition is a full set of ritualised procedures, undertaken in order to build a connection with the past. In their perspective, tradition is not something that has been left with predecessors but is instead 'invented' by people in the present. People employ 'traditional' materials to create new traditions according to certain social needs that exist in the current reality. Such traditions are invented through a set of complicated languages symbolising communication and practices. According to Jing (1996), tradition contains ritual meaning and attempts to reaffirm certain values and regulations; it has to be perceived to be continuous with the past. For Foucault, such invented traditions resonate with his claim that history is disrupted, but not continuous (Foucault, 1970b). Hobsbawm and Ranger (1983) claimed that those traditions that appeared to be ancient often instead originated quite close in time to their identification. In its own way, tradition could be invented rapidly, and thereby came into being non-linearly (Jing, 1996). Such tradition reflected a disruption from the past and perhaps the future as well. Invented tradition symbolises the way to respond to the new context according to the (constructed) old one.

This theorising about the idea of tradition is a reminder of influential French philosopher Maurice Halbwachs' conceptualisation. From a more micro-level perspective, he explained the internal drive for a society or a group of people to invent a tradition or a set of collective memories. He attempted to answer the question of why a society needs memory (Halbwachs, 1996). He argued that every individual holds an illusion that the current reality is somehow imperfect compared to the past. For example, older adults often romanticise their childhood and their twenties. Memory gives the past a scent of mystery and an illusion of perfection in another dimension (Halbwachs, 1995). The past is detached from the present. The past, formed through collective memory, is constrained from the present reality. In the present reality, relationships are often fixated. However, in the 'past' there were different types of people and relationships in which one has been embedded in different stages of life.

Only when the individual in the present is willing to accept or acknowledge various kinds of relationships in the past will these relationships appear influential in the past. These relationships do not constrain one as current relationships do (Luo, 2011). Therefore, Halbwachs (1996) contended that memories of the past are a way of escaping or an attempt to 'solve' the current reality. In the Chinese context, according to Luo (2011), just as individuals need memories to release current pressures and stresses, society needs collective memory to build a somewhat utopian view of 'the past' to express dissatisfactions about current inequalities and other social injustices. Such a utopia enables people to embellish, rectify, or moderate the past in their memory, in terms of the present (Luo, 2011). Just like tradition, collective memory is merely an invented discursive formation that aims to legitimate the connection between the past and the now.

The Great Leap Forward and Cultural Revolution Discursively Constructed as Taboo Topics. Taboo is a discursively constructed concept in Foucault's theories (Foucault, 1994). Foucault discussed taboos as constraints from subject, morality, and power majeure. In Foucault's view, people are forced to talk around taboo topics (Foucault, 1994). For instance, according to Xu (2007), people tended to use 'the past' (guoqu, 过去) or 'those years' (naxienian, 那些年) to avoid directly referring to the Great Leap Forward (GLF) and the Cultural Revolution (CR) because in China the GLF and CR are considered to be taboo topics. Since the Economic Reform in 1978, the GLF and CR have been discouraged from being deeply examined in the public discourse. According to Xu (2007), the 'scars' (trauma) caused by the GLF and CR only remain visible on the surface, without a clear indication of what lies beneath. He claimed that the political and public discourse had not conducted a thorough inquiry into that period of time, at least not that the public knows about. Rosen (2007) wrote about the GLF and CR collectively as a taboo topic from a Foucauldian discourse perspective. According to Manning and Wemheuer (2011), the government is reluctant to pay too much attention to events for which they bear responsibility.

It should be noted that from a Foucauldian theoretical perspective and from the perspective of the above authors, a taboo is not something upon which people can absolutely not remark but rather something that people do not have the complete freedom, consciously or subconsciously, to discuss or research. In vol. 1 of *The History of Sexuality*, Foucault explained that a taboo can be mentioned but is not encouraged to be discussed deeply due to stigmatisation and social rejection (Foucault, 1978c). In the Chinese political discourse, it is discouraged to place deep public criticism of the GLF and CR. In the public discourse, people are reluctant to remember a period of time that represents extensive and extreme hardship and struggle (Xu, 2007).

Agency and Change (Resistance). Foucault's discourse theory also explored means by which dominating discourses can be resisted and a form of agency can be practised. Discourse theory was criticised by both Giddens (1982) and Bourdieu (1991) for being too inclined to emphasise structure. For them, Foucault's discursive theory promotes discourse's predetermined focus on the subject in a capitalist society over the possibility of resistance against discursive hegemony and disciplinary force. According to Ouyang (2012), Foucault's discourse theory (in the early stage of Foucault's works) is more concerned with how discourse comes to (re)realise power relations through the production of knowledge and less with how people can make changes. Foucault's main focus was on how discourse generates knowledge and disciplines humanity through power relations and exercises. If everything is discourse, change can hardly be achieved. His criticism of current modernity and its disciplinary restrictions on humanity reached a dilemma that seems unresolvable; indeed, if everything is constructed through discourse and discursive power relations are everywhere, humanity has no way of escaping contextual structural forces (Foucault, 1980b).

However, in his later stage of life, Foucault appeared to be trying to search for a solution to this dilemma of the power of structure over agency through his theorising of *care of the self*, in which he drew on ancient Greek and Roman history of sexuality (Foucault, 2012a). He refuted the kind of accusation levelled by Giddens (1982) and later by Bourdieu (1991) and Ouyang (2012) in one of his interviews titled 'Truth, Power, Self: An Interview':

> How can you imagine that I think change is impossible, since what I have analyzed was always related to political action? All of *Discipline and Punish*

> is an attempt to answer this question and to show how a new way of thinking took place.... In my books I have really tried to ... show all the factors that interacted and the reactions of people. I believe in the freedom of people. To the same situation, people react in very different ways. (Foucault, 1988, p. 14)

In his two lectures at Dartmouth, Foucault talked about the legitimate possibility of agency of those who practise subjugated knowledge or those considered as subaltern groups who fail to meet the needs or interests of the dominant class (Foucault & Blasius, 1993). In my research, migrant peasant workers, who were misconceived and marginalised, are also considered capable of making sense of different discourses and power relations.

Although to a somewhat limited extent, Foucault did mention some modes of practice through which structural changes could take place. For example, *aesthetics of existence* is a passive technique, to an extent, in which the subject adopts natural and physical enjoyments to resist discursive hegemony, in an aesthetic of the self. Scholars such as Stuart Hall tried to develop ways of resistance to the dominant discourse, starting from Foucault's theory of aesthetics of existence (Hall, 1997). In his later work Foucault identified this stance with the activity of *parrhesia* or truth-telling (Foucault, 1999). The Foucauldian concept of parrhesia is commonly rendered not merely as truthful speech but as fearless speech (He & van Heugten, 2020). A key element of the concept, as described by Foucault, is that the undertaking to speak truth must represent some kind of existential risk for the speaker, who has some personal incentive not to speak the truth. In Chapters 8 and 9, parrhesia will be discussed as a possible way of achieving agency (change) or as a 'solution' for the current unsettling nature of the discursive construction of filial piety.

In my work, the agency starts from exploring and identifying different discourses of filial piety, rather than from jumping forward to locating the technological means for resistance at an epistemological level. As Foucault said, in his interview on 'An Aesthetics of Existence',

> One did not suggest what people ought to be, what they ought to do, what they ought to think and believe. It was a matter of showing how social mechanisms up to now have been able to work ... and then, starting from there, one left to the people themselves, knowing all the above, the possibility of self-determination and the choice of their own existence. (Foucault, 1977b, p. 50)

Hence, as Foucault noted, it is meaningful to first identify various mechanisms involved in discourses of filial piety in order to make sense of participants' constructed selves. Only through this process will participants be able to practise some of the techniques of the self that Foucault mentioned in his works.

Power and Governmental Discourse

Foucault's perspective on power can be contrasted to conflict theorist and functionalist views of power which mainly refer to different understandings of domination (Gaventa, 2003). On the one hand, many conflict theorists see power as a means to fulfilling one's goal. On the other hand, most functionalists consider power as a collective trait. The first perspective views domination as individual actors' ability to reach their goal. However, this perspective does not explain power's structural features. The latter perspective views domination as a structural feature of the social system. Structure determines power completely, and power breaks away from agentive actions. The two perspectives can be employed together in an attempt to explain complementary relationships.

According to Gaventa (2003), Foucault built his theory on power. His work represented a radical departure from previous perspectives on power that essentialised a pyramid-shaped power structure (Gaventa, 2003; Sheridan & Foucault, 1980). Foucault saw power as enacted and embodied rather than possessed, diffuse rather than concentrated (Foucault, 2008). For him, power does not come from A forcing B to do something but from interaction with discourse.

> Power is everywhere: not because it embraces everything, but because it comes from everywhere. Power is not an institution, nor a structure, nor a possession. It is the name we give to a complex strategic situation in a particular society. (Foucault, 1978c, p. 93)

Foucault claimed that in modern society, power operates through a series of techniques involving subjecting to knowledge, making visible, ordering, normalising, and disciplining. Just as discourse is embedded in every aspect of our society, power is everywhere (Oliver, 2010). Power is not only about negative influences such as suppressing, oppression, inspection, separation, hiding, and so on, but also actively produces reality and rituals for 'truth' (Fendler, 2010). Foucault expressed neutrality in relation to the nature of power by also focusing on its productive and positive side (Foucault, 1978b).

In Foucault's time, the philosophical and sociological focus was shifted from structural political economy towards culture (Ouyang, 2012). Foucault has been criticised by scholars, especially post-Marxists, for his neglect of macro-level power relations in society (Daldal, 2014). Many post-Marxists even borrowed his idea of *bio-power* and *power/knowledge* to complement the framework of cultural hegemony (Gaventa, 2003). Marxists have given a more systematic explanation of society on the macro level. For them, class conflicts and a nation-state's powerful position are the essential matters. However, for Foucault, government is only one of all power relationships, important but not uniquely so. In modernity, power is exercised everywhere and is intractable (Foucault, 1970b). Although he did not dwell on this, Foucault himself did embrace the idea that apparatus and institutions matter a lot. That is to say, although power becomes more broad and hidden in the modern era, governmental power relations are still very important (Foucault, 2007).

The Chinese government's policies highly influenced the (re)construction and (re)production of filial piety in China. According to Huang (2011), modernity is a process of reconstructing our everyday life to be a part of the modern world, and Chinese modernity is propelled predominantly by the state. She thought that the state's exercise of power over the reproduction of filial piety included two main policies: the one-child policy, and the replacement of burial with cremation. The one-child policy conflicted with the notion of traditional filial piety that held that being fruitful by having a significant number of children is the most important filial responsibility (Luo, 2013). In addition, the government forbids traditional burial rituals, which, to a great extent, diminishes the spiritual authority of ancestors and parents (Huang, 2011). These examples represent an extreme form of disciplinary power (Foucault, 1970b). According to Foucault (1991), the ultimate goal of the modern state is to regulate the population for economic reasons. Therefore, a Foucauldian discourse analysis needs to take careful account of the institutional power relations of the state which may not, on the surface, appear economic. And clearly, given the state's far-reaching authority, this is also important in the Chinese context.

Yan (2006) proposed that there are two main perspectives on how the Chinese state's exercise of power has influenced filial piety. On the one hand, after the foundation of the People's Republic of China, the socialist revolution diminished the social foundation of filial piety, which included the patriarchal clan system, ancestral beliefs, and family-owned property. Moreover, neoliberal market economic reform also weakened these foundational mechanisms. A new rational intergenerational relation replaced the traditional filial piety. On the other hand, according to Davis-Friedmann (1991), China did not yet have enough resources to build a comprehensive welfare system. Therefore, it continued to rely on Confucian filial piety to maintain social order and sustainable intergenerational relationships. These two different views on interactions between the state and filial piety represent a top-down approach to analysing these relationships. My research took a bottom-up approach, involving an exploration of how my participants viewed their own (re)construction of filial piety in interaction with the state's influence.

Archaeology and Genealogy

Crowley (2009) described Foucault's 'archaeology' and 'genealogy' as 'two halves of a complementary approach, alternating and supporting each other' (p. 341). Foucault's concept of archaeology may be best represented in his earlier work on the specific constructions of social discourse on madness, health, and the history of ideas in *Madness and Civilization*, *The Birth of the Clinic*, and *The Order of Things*, and particularly in his methodological treatise, *The Archaeology of Knowledge*. During the 1970s, he used genealogy to replace archaeology. Simplistically speaking, genealogy adopted power into the picture of archaeology to a greater extent (Foucault, 1978a).

In *The Archaeology of Knowledge*, Foucault described the 'archive' as 'a practice that causes a multiplicity of statements to emerge as so many regular events, as so many things to be dealt with and manipulated' (Foucault, 1970a, p. 130). In this way, Foucault conceptualised a field in which discourses take place in and around a given empirical set of regularities that can be generated by any contingent set of historical circumstances, and that may limit or distinguish one discourse from another. In confronting this givenness, Foucault noted,

> [Archaeology] does not imply the search for a beginning ... it deprives us of our continuities ... it breaks the thread of transcendental teleologies ... [rather it] questions the already-said at the element of its existence....

> Archaeology describes discourses [simply] as practices specified in the elements of the archive. (Foucault, 1970a, p. 131)

In his essay 'Nietzsche, Genealogy, History', Foucault (1978a) defined genealogy as

> [requiring] patience and a knowledge of details, and [depending] on a vast accumulation of source material … In short, genealogy demands relentless erudition. Genealogy does not oppose itself to history as the lofty and profound gaze of the philosopher might compare to the molelike perspective of the scholar; on the contrary, it rejects the metahistorical deployment of ideal significations … It opposes itself to the search for 'origins'. (Foucault, 1978a, pp. 78–90)

From Vol. 1 of *the History of Sexuality* and his interview 'The Confession of the Flesh', Foucault's genealogical debate became more political and more focused on the relationship between practice and discourse. His analysis of knowledge also became more related to power (Foucault, 1972b, 1978c).

Both archaeology and genealogy are useful for critiquing the construction of a linear history of filial piety. In my analysis of Chinese filial piety I also incorporated a consideration of the Chinese Confucian and neo-Confucian traditions, as well as drawing on various nineteenth- and twentieth-century efforts to criticise these Chinese traditions, as noted in Chapter 2. I also addressed post-economic reform (1978) social policies in China, that attempt to compensate for the challenges that industrialisation, modernisation, and internal migration have placed on the support of elderly parents by their children. My analysis included sufficient historical inquiry to describe the evolution of these elements of the archive within which the discourse took place. I have not attempted to define the discourse as some sort of derived reflection or consequence of those elements. This reflects my scepticism about the epistemic certainty of such a causal relationship, in keeping with Foucault's claim that history is broken and non-linear (Foucault, 1978a). It is also, in part, simply a reflection of my greater interest in the subjective significance of the discourse itself.

Subjectivity, Genealogy, and Discourse of Filial Piety

The question of subjectivity arose in Foucault's work after his deployment of the concept of genealogy. In contrast to archaeology, Foucauldian genealogy more directly explored the ways that social forces exercise power over individual subjectivities, in part by direct and intensive efforts to construct the knowledge of people in society. The classic Foucauldian example is the creation of the surveillance state, described in *Discipline and Punish* (Foucault & Sheridan, 1977). Foucault argued that the transformation of punishment from public spectacle to incarceration puts inspection, observation, direction, and self-examination at the centre of the idea of corrective punishment. But the greater significance of this change is that it was reflected in the state's attitude towards its own citizens as well—the spread of 'surveillance, control and policing' as a strategy through which most social institutions collaborated in efforts to discipline the general public, in support of the interests of leading economic forces (Crowley, 2009, p. 342). The goal of the exercise of power is 'the formation of subjectivity' (Crowley, 2009, p. 343).

> [T]hrough the control of ideas [the state and institutions] reconstructs its subjects to produce new actions, habits and skills and ultimately new kinds of people ... Discipline and surveillance is interiorized to the point that each individual is his or her own overseer. (Crowley, 2009, p. 434)

Such a description of the genealogy of subjectivities obviously sets the agenda for a critical analysis of discourse to explore the formation of subjectivity by power, and to explore ways that subjects can engage in that discourse to resist the self-interested agendas of power. Such an analysis assumes that the subject's goal is to reassert their own autonomy and to exercise self-care. Yet this very dramatic description of the interaction of power and subjective knowledge seems an exaggeration employed for rhetorical effect. Foucault himself, in 'Two Lectures [on Power and Knowledge]' (Foucault, 1980b), seemed to restate the issue more mildly when he spoke of 'a sense of the increasing vulnerability to criticism of things, institutions, practices, discourses', to which he hoped he had contributed (Foucault, 1980b, p. 80).

In opposition to globalising and totalising styles of thinking, Foucault (1980a) proposed criticism of a 'local character', emphasising a 'return of knowledge', especially of 'subjugated knowledges' (p. 81), which include 'naive knowledge', 'popular knowledges', and the 'disqualified' voices of disadvantaged groups of people (migrant peasant workers in this research). Research focusing on genealogy can attempt to recover and reconstruct these knowledges, allowing them to emerge from their suppression by more institutionalised forms of knowledge (p. 83). Such research will pay greater attention to the voices of 'speaking, discoursing subjects' (p. 85) and, without asserting any positive value for ignorance or mindlessness, will more carefully ask questions about whether it makes sense to 'diminish' or 'disqualify' particular voices just because they are not associated with hierarchies of power (Foucault, 1980a, p. 85).

Within the context of Chinese filial piety discourse, a sensitivity to genealogies of knowledge enables me to look at the interaction between power and knowledge without making oversimplified assumptions about the binding or normative force of particular traditional concepts. For instance, in invoking Confucian values, the tradition itself is ambiguous. Classic Confucianism emphasises broad concepts of 'respect' and 'care' without extensive normative elaboration. In the later neo-Confucian tradition, Confucian concepts of filial piety are elaborated in prescriptive detail and backed by an explicitly and implicitly authoritarian intention. However, that is not to say the traits of these two discourses do not overlap. The difference can only be simplified for the sake of understanding.

Disciplinary Power of Neo-Confucianism

I consider how neo-Confucian filial discourse resembles a western modern space where (scientific) disciplinary power is practised and exercised, as Foucault described in his books *The Archaeology of Knowledge* and *The Order of Things: An Archaeology of the Human Sciences* (Foucault, 1970a, 1970b). As discussed in Chapter 2, the teaching of Confucius himself (over 2,000 years ago) was different from neo-Confucianism (dominating Chinese society from the twelfth century to the eighteenth century). Ancient Confucianism valued 'respect' and 'care' for parents. It did not exact so many requirements of children, such as to obey parents and other people, including the emperor. By contrast, neo-Confucianism placed a great many restrictions on individuals. In the neo-Confucian discourse of filial piety, the 'obedience' principle was the main constituent of children's relationship with both parents and the emperor. The provision of care and intergenerational emotional bonds ranked below the principle of having to 'obey'. Neo-Confucianists elevated filial morality onto the 'truth' level, which they called the *li* (principle). *Li* referred to the ways in which everything in the world comes into being; according to *li*, filial morality existed before human existence and human society. Filial rules and regulations became almost 'disciplinary', akin to how Foucault described modern disciplinary science.

Apart from the contextual and social difference between China at that time (where there were no modern scientific disciplines after neo-Confucianism's founding and before the eighteenth century) and western modern society, there are other differences in terms of the nature of this disciplinary power. An example of a disciplinary form of power in the Foucauldian sense is located at the beginning of western modernisation when religious forms of control lost their dominance to scientific disciplines. However, during the Song dynasty in China, religions such as Zen Buddhism and Taoism never dominated Chinese society as Christianity did in the west during the pre-modern era. Instead, the ubiquitous feature of modern 'disciplinary' discursive power in Foucault's writing appears to parallel neo-Confucian discourse, which is everywhere.

Another similarity between disciplinary modernity and neo-Confucianism is that both have experienced criticism. Modernity has been heavily criticised by Foucault and Foucauldian discourse analysts. In China, neo-Confucianism was already heavily criticised at the beginning of nineteenth century and during CR. However, there are two different opinions about the critiques of CR. One opinion holds that filial piety (especially in neo-Confucianism) was completely criticised during CR (Zhang, 2017). On the other hand, there are some scholars who have expressed the belief that rejection of filial piety only applied at the level of the family. Filial piety towards the state (which used to be the emperor) did not face criticism, but instead was further reinforced (consider, for example, the national worship of Chairman Mao). That is to say, the 'disciplinary' power of state filial piety still prevailed during CR, despite filial piety being overtly criticised at the level of the family.

In the wake of rising political and public discourse of promoting filial piety in recent years, as mentioned in Chapter 2, the disciplinary power of filial discourse may re-enter Chinese people's everyday life and awareness. However, obedience is a far more prominent concept in neo-Confucian than in classical Confucian tradition. Since obedience to parents is not as prominent a feature of contemporary discourses of filial piety, the oppressive nature of filial piety may not be as strong as western modern scientific disciplinary power. That is to say, to some extent, the current circumstance of blending between alleged western modernity and Chinese traditions might have already enabled a hidden resistance to the disciplinary power of filial discourse, at least to some extent. However, by contrast to the requirement to obey parents, the obligation to obey the government is still relatively strong, which could potentially enforce the disciplinary power of filial piety. In that case, Foucault's strategy for resisting western modernity could be useful for the Chinese current context, in terms of magnifying the care and respect aspects of filial discourse, instead of emphasising blind obedience.

Foucault and Chinese Philosophies

Foucault's theories are useful for research on filial piety and family care. In Chapter 3 I wrote about the challenges that scholars have to confront when they investigate Chinese matters using a western methodology. There are many differences between the Chinese and western context as well as their philosophical traditions. For instance, western philosophy has a focus on logical thinking and things that do not concern people's daily life, while Chinese philosophies have a major concern with action and practices in relation to people's daily life as well as related skills and ways of governing (Wang, 2010). However, Foucault criticised many western philosophical traditions of the modern era. His ideas bear many similarities to Chinese traditional philosophies, three of which will be explained in this section. Firstly, both share a tendency to address the complexity of power relations and the relational self. Secondly, both tend to value action/practice as opposed to placing emphasis on a search for the objective/universal truth for humanity. Lastly, both look back into ancient history to look for resources and possible solutions for current issues, such as a technique of *care of the self* (parrhesia/telling the truth, which will be discussed in Chapters 9 and 10).

Complexity of Relationality

While in many other western social theories, the conception of the self often assumes clear boundaries with others (and with the truth) philosophically (Barbalet, 2014), Foucault explored the complexity of the construction of the self through various power relations. As Foucault claimed that 'power relations are rooted in the whole network of the social' (Foucault, 2000, p. 345), the network of various power relations depreciates the distinction between the self and others, as the focus is on elements in interaction within relationships. According to Foucault (2000), social phenomena and the social construction of these phenomena should not be studied as separate objects, but as connectedness scrutinised through an exploration of the interactions of people, concepts, and things. From a Foucauldian perspective, relationships resemble a network of human and contextual interactions (Foucault, 1980b).

In the ancient Chinese context, Confucian relations assume set ethical and moral rules of teacher–student, parent–child, husband–wife, ruler–ruled relationships as relational subject interactions (Canda, 2013). Filial piety is derived from this relational self. This relational concept of the self resonates with the understanding of the dynamics of yin/yang (Hodder, 2000). The yin/yang diagram suggests its relational nature (yin in the yang and yang in the yin). For example, a son is characterised as yin to his parents but yang to his wife and children. This fluidity and relativity of yin/yang accentuates the importance of social relations in the formation of the self. This formation is not established through internal predispositions but through external relations (Lin, 2013). The self only exists through interactions with others. In many Chinese philosophies, the formation of the self is a process of positioning and identification within a complex of social relations rather than an ascribed collective entity (Lin, 2013). The fulfilment of one's social roles is inextricably involved in the formation of self-identity in a Chinese context.

Drawing on this convergence of ideas about the relationality of the self, Chinese scholar Shen (2012) developed a theory incorporating both Chinese philosophical tradition and discourse theory to research intercultural issues. Shen wrote:

> On the linguistic level, one should translate one's ideas or propositions into a language understandable to others. On the pragmatic level, one should draw one's own ideas and values out from one's world and then put them into other people's world to see whether they are valid there. On the ontological level, one should strive for a direct experience with reality itself, such as a person, a community, or the ultimate reality, in order to have access to the different world of others. (Shen, 2012, p. 181)

The various relations in which people are involved and that involve people in society form a complicated chaos that becomes very difficult to unpack and explain. Akin to Foucault's example of psychiatric discourse, the discourse of filial piety does not only include the different responsibilities of being a filial son, daughter, and daughter-in-law, parents' position and authority, intergenerational relationships, and so on, but also includes how filial discourse interacts with social institutions and practices that do not belong to the obvious filial discourse. The subjective position and the notion of 'the self' are created through these salient and hidden relationships (Foucault & Khalfa, 2009). In his explanation of *madness*, Foucault identified many different relationships among different shareholders, such as policymakers, psychiatrists, family members, and psychiatric institutions. Psychiatric discourse offers a formulated regulation that creates certain power and body relations to settle the seemingly chaotic relationships. For Foucault, all of the questions he talked about in *The Order of Things: An Archaeology of the Human Sciences* were related to power relations (Foucault, 1972b). As discourse is where power takes place, different discourses create and are generated from relevant power relations and exercises. The discourse of filial piety allows different power exercises to unfold in unique ways for migrant peasant workers. In return, the discourse is also more complex because it incorporates a series of mechanisms for power relations.

Current Chinese society is facing rapid structural change as a result of both global and domestic drivers. Such drivers stimulate extreme comparisons that contrast renovation with an attempt to remain unchanged and permanent (Xian, 2013). The power relations constructed around these two directional comparisons are bound to be of much greater complexity than dualistic contrasts can adequately reflect.

The Pragmatic Nature of Chinese Philosophies and Foucault

Foucault paid a great deal of attention to practice, especially in the later stage of his life. Many influential western philosophers have had an overwhelming interest in language in relation to its role in human society. For example, Heidegger pointed out that existence and being forms language, and language also forms existence and being (Kockelmans, 1972). In his early published books, such as the *Archaeology of Knowledge* and *Discipline and Punish,* Foucault focused on the omnipresence of discourse; almost everything is created through discursive formation. However, his definition of discourse was not restricted to language. For example, Willig (2008) developed six stages for Foucauldian discourse analysis, based on Foucault's discourse theory. In the fifth stage, she focused on practice and its relationship with discourse in terms of the limitations and possibilities of discursive action. Her practice step was built on Foucault's definition and explanation of discourse and power. In Foucault's vision, practice and social interactions are disciplined by power, and power is regulated and generated by discourse (Foucault, 1972a, 2000). In Foucault's (2012a, 2012b; 1998) three volumes of *The History of Sexuality*, he shifts from the discussion of a discursively constructed self to that of care of the self or cultivation of the self through technologies of the self (e.g., meditation, telling the truth/*parrhesia*). He argues that the self also contains agency and freedom through a set of practices, which he retrieves from ancient Greek and Roman times.

Cai (2005) and Feng (1995) thought Chinese philosophers did not write many theoretical books, mainly because of the Chinese emphasis on valuing action/practice. As also discussed in Chapter 3, Chinese philosophies had a tradition of focus on action/practice, including Confucianism, Taoism, and Zen Buddhism. For example, there is a well-known saying from the *Zuozhuan*, an ancient historical narrative that documents an ancient historical chronicle of the Spring and Autumn Periods (ca. 771–ca. 476 BCE, also the time of Confucius and Laozi): '太上有立德, 其次有立功, 其次有立言' (The first step is to set one's virtue; the second step is to set one's meritorious conduct; the third step is to expand one's ideas in writing) (Feng, 1995, p. 8). Chinese philosophers believed the ultimate goal was to nurture one's inner virtue and contribute to societal governing in the external world, i.e., set one's meritorious conduct (Feng, 1995). To write about one's theories and ideas was the last step on a pathway (Feng, 1995). Therefore, Chinese philosophical books were often written by the specific Chinese philosopher's followers; moreover, the writings were mostly an aggregation of a philosopher's notes and daily conversations (Cai, 2005). Feng (1995) surmised that it was because the ancient Chinese used bamboo slips as paper to write, a medium that is heavy and inconvenient, that Chinese philosophical writings were so short. They mostly consisted of sharp, to-the-point conclusions with little argumentation and few illustrations or demonstrations (Feng, 1995). This later became a tradition or fashion in writing style. Feng (1995) admitted that Chinese philosophers' written language was not so logical or clear as a result, but also pointed to the infinite possibilities opened up by Chinese philosophical indications which were a result of exactly these illogical and unclear features.

In ancient Chinese philosophy (especially in the pre-Qin dynasty, before 221 BCE), knowledge is realised through actions (Song, 2008) rather than through language and learning. Confucius (551–479 BCE) once said that studying the *Book of Poems* develops the practice of governing (Song, 2008). Another Confucianist, Xunzi (ca. 336–ca. 236 BCE) also stated that knowing cannot compare to action/practice (Duperon, 2017). Taoists also valued action, although many have claimed they do not (Bender, 2016). One of Laozi's most famous quotes is *zhidaguorupengxiaoxian* (治大国如烹小鲜, to govern a big country is the same as slowly cooking a small pot of stew or stir-fry) (Bender, 2016). It means the right amount of governance is crucial. Taoism did not dwell on the importance of language in terms of articulating 'Tao' (the way) but rather represented 'Tao' through actions (Bender, 2016). Of course, there were stages, especially during the Han dynasty (202 BCE–220 CE), when knowing was valued and the importance of action/practices was neglected (Song, 2008). Some scholars, such as the famous Han dynasty Confucianist Dongzhongshu (179–104 BCE), did not care about anything but to obtain knowledge from books. However, Song (2008) claimed that the mainstream Chinese philosophers deemed action/practice as of primary importance throughout Chinese philosophical history. Zen Buddhism (originating in China) also valued action/practice; for example, monks developed kung fu as a way of becoming Buddha. They valued this much more than meditation and chanting, differing in this from Indian Buddhists (Ladany et al., 2013). The famous Zen Master Mazu Daoyi (709–788 CE) once taught that the only way to become a Buddha is to do deeds, instead of only studying Buddhist books and meditations (Ladany et al., 2013).

This is not to say knowing is not important. After the time of the above-mentioned Chinese philosophers, different neo-Confucianists (the school of neo-Confucianism is thought to have formed after ca. 960 CE) argued about the knowledge and action interface for many years. At first, the Cheng brothers (Cheng Yi 1033–1107, Cheng Jing 1032–1085) claimed that knowledge comes before action/practice. Without knowing how, one cannot carry out appropriate actions (Tucker, 1991). Then their student Zhu Xi (1130–1200) developed their theory with a different angle. Zhu thought action/practice is more important than knowing

(Tucker, 1991). Another neo-Confucianist, Wang Yangming (1472–1529), built on the Cheng brothers' and Zhu Xi's ideas and made his own epistemological argument, namely that knowing and action/practice are one and the same (Tu, 1976). However, later Wang's theory evolved into an argument that only knowing is meaningful within the knowing/action interface (Tu, 1976). If these two are the same, one can replace the other one. Wang's followers ended up only valuing knowledge (Song, 2008). It was not until over 100 years later when another philosopher, Wang Fuzi (1619–1692), argued against such a view and developed the newest theoretical construction of knowing/action (Song, 2008). For him, action came first, before knowledge; action and practice could carry knowledge; knowledge, however, cannot carry action and practice (Song, 2013).

Therefore, there is substantial and solid common ground between the pragmatic nature of Foucault's discourse theory and filial piety. Foucault's theories provide an appropriate theoretical fit for my research.

Looking Back and Care of the Self

There is third similarity between Chinese theory and practice and Foucauldian theory and practice which involves looking back to ancient times and history for resources and theoretical foundations on which to base critiques of contemporary discourses. Many ancient Chinese philosophies, including Confucianism and Taoism, criticise the concept of progress and argue that the 'best' times in human society lie in the ancient past. Foucault also had a tendency to delve back into ancient history for more enlightenment and possible next steps to support his criticisms of modernity.

Foucault, by comparing how sexuality is constructed differently in the modern era and in ancient Greek and Roman times, tried to find a solution to break the constraints of disciplinary power within modernity. In *The History of Sexuality II* and *III*, Foucault (2012a, 2012b) explained that in modern society, the lustful self is constructed through Christianity, psychology, psychiatry, health science, and other disciplinary surveillance and regulation. The lustful self is a subjectified object which appears to be free-willed (Foucault, 2012b). However, this objectified free subject is not free (Foucault, 2012a). In his first volume of *The History of Sexuality*, Foucault (1978b) explained that sexuality comprehensively governs humanity through discursively constructed scientific truths about sexuality. No free subject can be practised under such discursive construction

(Foucault, 1978b). In the second volume, he discovered that there was an ethical practice by free subjects in the ancient Greek and Roman period (Foucault, 2012a). For Foucault, individuals in ancient times had the freedom to practice sexuality through their 'natural' sense of pleasure, as opposed to through social constructions, such as 'lust' and 'desire'. In other words, they were not yet constrained by socially constructed ideas of lust and desire. In his lecture on *The Hermeneutics of the Subject* in 1982, he clearly pointed out that free subjects can only be reached through *epimeleia heautou* (care of the self) (Foucault, 2005).

In Foucault's later life, philosophy as a way of life, different from the previous dominant philosophical discourse that separated philosophy as a reflexive thought from philosophers' personalities and lives, became an academic trend (Hadot, 1995). According to Hadot (1995), the ancient Greek and Roman philosophies, with which Foucault was fascinated, also belong to the form of philosophy that views itself as a way of life. Care of the self refers to a form of practice that one can adopt as a means to cultivating oneself (Foucault, 2005). This too shares common ground with Chinese philosophies. Confucianism is a rich source for cultivation of the self (Cheng, 2004). In his lecture on ''Technologies of the Self', Foucault talked about the ways of care of the self in ancient Greek and Roman times. This resonates with his ethics theory in *The History of Sexuality,* which is not only a theory but also a regulation of actions and behaviours, a practice of the self, a way of life, or aesthetics of existence. Care of the self deals with a sense of change and free will and ability to effect change in the dominant discourse.

Foucault's critique of modernity and his care of the self-theory raised the question of returning to the ethical subject of ancient times. Foucault adopted the concept of ethics to make sense of the free subject (Foucault, 2005). Ethics refers to the relationship between one and oneself and is different from morality in Foucault's definition (Foucault, 2012a). The essence of ethics lies in freedom of practice (Foucault, 2005). In ancient Greek and Roman times, the intensity of dominant power relations, the will for truth, the regulation of self-surveillance and self-discipline, and the degree of objectification of the subject remained at a low level and represented an ethical goal of care of the self. Therefore, subjects were able to be free to practice at that time. He asserted that there was a rupture in the history of the relationship between subject and truth. This rupture was called the Cartesian moment (when the subject's own mind becomes an object of knowledge and discourse in western philosophy;

Foucault, 2005). Before the Cartesian moment, knowing oneself was always associated with taking care of oneself. After the Cartesian moment, these elements are no longer associated, and knowledge is not related to subject or ethical requirements, but only to disciplinary power and discursive knowledge. The subject of modernity becomes a rational self-knowing subject reliant on scientific disciplinary knowledge and discourse, but not an ethical care of the self subject (Foucault, 2005).

Filial subject practice was also constrained by external disciplinary forces (based on extreme interpretations of Confucian classical books and neo-Confucian theories, imperial filial governing, etc.). However, the main content for classical Confucianism was a course of construction of the ethical self (free subject). For example, in ancient times, especially before neo-Confucianism (first constructed in the eighth century), it was one of the filial duties for children to correct their parents if parents were wrong. In classic Confucianism, the filial self can be cultivated through ways of practice for each individual. That is to say, filial piety, at least potentially, does not only contain features of modernity, which produce discursive subjects through disciplinary power relations, but also ethical features, which provide means to gaining freedom of practice through care of the self. I argue that both features of classic Confucian discourse and neo-Confucian discourse of filial piety exist in contemporary Chinese society, even though the disciplinary discursive formation might be dominating.

According to C. Wang (2016), Confucianism constructs the ethical self mainly through edification (*jiaohua* 教化). Edification refers to self-transformation through studying Confucian books or enabling transformation through teaching others from Confucian books (C. Wang, 2016). C. Wang (2016) thought that individuals who acquired or were taught edification all had the ability to complete ethical self-transformation, especially before neo-Confucianism. As noted in Chapter 2, during this time even children were believed able to consider ethical implications and were allowed to point out and correct parents' unethical behaviours and thoughts. Filial piety also extended to the relationship between the emperor (as the father) and his subjects (as the son), and like any children, Confucianists were able to rebel against the emperor because they had freedom of practice (D. Wang, 2016). They had a series of techniques of care of the self, such as reflexive interpretation of the Confucian classical books, Confucian rituals, and so on (D. Wang, 2016). These means of cultivation of the self, such as meditation and talking to oneself, resonate with Foucault's suggestions for techniques of care of the self.

The will to search for truth and oppressive disciplinary force were both strengthened after the foundation of neo-Confucianism, from the eighth century in China. In the Chinese context, the ethical subject was much freer before the eightheighth century. As explained in Chapter 2, neo-Confucianism created a somewhat disciplinary knowledge of filial piety and filial practice. Neo-Confucian regulation and rules of filial piety became the truth for Chinese people. Westernisation since the New Culture Movement (1910s and 1920s) cultivated another form of disciplinary power relation, which also potentially weakened the oppressive power of the neo-Confucian discourse of filial piety. However, the complexity generated through the confrontation of two forms of disciplinary discursive power also created confusion and uncertainty for cultural norms such as filial piety, which the west did not have to face during its transition to modernity. This confusion and uncertainty could add to the neoliberal unsettledness and become uncontrollable.

Conversely, however, such confusion and uncertainty may also open a window for a search for the ethical subject, reaching back into the ancient history of China. If we look at the historical trajectory of western philosophy, it (simplistically put) went through stages from the ancient Greek and Roman period, to Christianity, to modernity and modern science. On the other hand, in China the historical trajectory of philosophy moved from the classical Confucian period, to the neo-Confucian period, to modernity and modern times. There are some similarities in terms of what has been discussed above about care of the self and discursive domination. However, in the Chinese context, modernity was not an exact match with western modernity, and care of the filial self and its technologies might still linger (including because of the extreme criticism of the neo-Confucian discourse of filial piety that arose during the GLF and the CR). Whether viewed as a potential window of opportunity to act with an agency or as a problem with a lack of clear solution, there is an urgent need to examine the discourse of filial piety in contemporary Chinese society in order to identify conditions and mechanisms that may affect its practice in current and future generations.

Conclusion

Foucault's discourse theory is meaningful for my research not just because I also have a need for a theoretical approach that enables me to critique the disciplinary discursive power relations existing both in modern western and in Chinese society. Foucault's theories on power and truth have an important similarity with Chinese philosophies in that they recognise the complexity of relationality. Within the discourse of filial piety, the selves that individuals construct are as relational as power relations in the Foucauldian sense. Chinese philosophies (which highlight the importance of filial piety) incorporate a pragmatic feature, just as Foucault did, especially in the latter stage of his life. In his later life, Foucault moved on from a discursive subjectivity to a subjectivity with a possibility of change or agency. He reiterated care of the self (technologies of the self) from ancient Greek and Roman times, which resonates with the Chinese philosophical tradition of criticising progress and highly valuing the past. Based on the above discussion, there are solid grounds for combining Foucault's discourse theory with Chinese philosophies when it comes to examining an issue that is part of the essence of many Chinese philosophies: filial piety.

References

Barbalet, J. (2014). Greater self, lesser self: Dimensions of self-interest in Chinese filial piety. *Journal for the Theory of Social Behaviour, 44*(2), 186–205. https://doi.org/10.1111/jtsb.12037

Bender, J. (2016). Justice as the practice of non-coercive action: A study of John Dewey and classical Daoism. *Asian Philosophy, 26*(1), 20–37. https://doi.org/10.1080/09552367.2015.1136200

Bourdieu, P. (1991). The peculiar history of scientific reason. *Sociological Forum, 6*(1), 3–26. https://doi.org/10.1007/BF01112725

Cai, W. (2005). An essay on Feng Youlan's view on Chinese philosophy: In commemoration of Feng Youlan's 100th birth year 论冯友兰的中国哲学观——纪念冯友兰先生诞辰 110 周年. *Henan Normal University Press: Philosophy and Social Science 河南师范大学学报: 哲学社会科学版, 32*(1), 1–6.

Canda, E. R. (2013). Filial piety and care for elders: A contested Confucian virtue reexamined. *Journal of Ethnic and Cultural Diversity in Social Work, 22*(3–4), 213–234. https://doi.org/10.1080/15313204.2013.843134

Cheng, C. (2004). A theory of Confucian selfhood: Self-cultivation and free will in Confucian philosophy. *Frontiers of Philosophy in China, 2*(4), 547–556. https://link.springer.com/journal/11466

Crowley, Ú. (2009). Genealogy method. In R. Kitchin & N. Thrift (Eds.), *International encyclopedia of human geography* (pp. 341–344). Elsevier.

Daldal, A. (2014). Power and ideology in Michel Foucault and Antonio Gramsci: A comparative analysis. *Review of History and Political Science* (2), 149–167. https://www.annualreviews.org/journal/polisci

Davis-Friedmann, D. (1991). *Long lives: Chinese elderly and the communist revolution*. Stanford University Press.

Dreyfus, H. L., & Rabinow, P. (1982). *Michel Foucault: Beyond structuralism and hermeneutics*. University of Chicago Press.

Duperon, M. (2017). Solving for the triad: Xunzi and Wendell Berry on sustainable agriculture as ethical practice. *Philosophy East and West, 67*(2), 380–398. https://doi.org/10.1353/pew.2017.0031

Edwards, D. (2013). Naturalness, representation and the metaphysics of truth. *European Journal of Philosophy, 21*(3), 384–401. https://doi.org/10.1111/j.1468-0378.2011.00452.x

Fendler, L. (2010). *Michel Foucault* (Vol. 22). Continuum.

Feng, Y. (1995). *History of Chinese philosophy中国哲学史*. Zhonghua Shuju.

Foucault, M. (1970). *The archaeology of knowledge*. Tavistock.

Foucault, M. (1970). *The order of things: An archaeology of the human sciences*. Tavistock.

Foucault, M. (1972a). *The archaeology of knowledge: And the discourse on language*. Pantheon.

Foucault, M. (1972b). The confession of the flesh. In C. Gordon (Ed.), *Power/knowledge: Selected interviews and other writings 1972–1977* (pp. 194–228). Pantheon.

Foucault, M. (1977a). Truth and power. In C. Gordon (Ed.), *Power/knowledge: Selected interviews and other writings 1972–1977* (pp. 109–133). Pantheon.

Foucault, M. (1977). An aesthetics of existence. In L. D. Kritzman (Ed.), *Politics, philosophy, culture: Interviews and other writings, 1984* (pp. 47–53). Routledge.

Foucault, M. (1978a). Nietzsche, genealogy, history. *Semiotexte, 3*(1), 78–94.

Foucault, M. (1978b). *The history of sexuality* (1st US ed.). Pantheon.

Foucault, M. (1978c). *The history of sexuality* (vol. 1). Vintage.

Foucault, M. (1980). *Language, counter-memory, practice: Selected essays and interviews*. Blackwell.

Foucault, M. (1980b). *Power/knowledge: Selected interviews and other writings, 1972–1977*. Pantheon.

Foucault, M. (1988). *Truth, power, self: An interview paper presented at Technologies of the Self: A seminar with Michel Foucault*. Tavistock.

Foucault, M. (1991). *The Foucault effect: Studies in governmentality*. University of Chicago Press.
Foucault, M. (1994). *The selected work of Foucault 福柯集*. Shanghai Fareast.
Foucault, M. (1998). *The history of sexuality (vol. 1): The will to knowledge* (R. Hurley, Trans.). Penguin.
Foucault, M. (1999). *Discourse and truth: The problematization of parrhesia; Six lectures given by Michel Foucault at the University of California at Berkeley, October–November 1983*. Retrieved from https://foucault.info
Foucault, M. (2000). *The subject and power* (J. D. Faubion, Ed.). The New Press.
Foucault, M. (2005). *The hermeneutics of the subject: Lectures at the Collège de France 1981–1982* (G. Burchell, Trans.). Picador.
Foucault, M. (2007). *Security, territory, population: Lectures at the Collège de France, 1977–78*. Springer.
Foucault, M. (2008). *The birth of biopolitics* (G. Burchell, Trans.). Palgrave Macmillan.
Foucault, M. (2012a). *The history of sexuality (vol. 2): The use of pleasure*. Vintage.
Foucault, M. (2012b). *The history of sexuality (vol. 3): The care of the self*. Vintage.
Foucault, M., & Blasius, M. (1993). About the beginning of the hermeneutics of the self: Two lectures at Dartmouth. *Political Theory, 21*(2), 198–227. https://doi.org/10.1177/0090591793021002004
Foucault, M., & Khalfa, J. (2009). *History of madness*. Routledge.
Foucault, M., & Sheridan, A. (1977). *Discipline and punish: The birth of the prison*. Penguin.
Gaventa, J. (2003). *Power after Lukes: An overview of theories of power since Lukes and their application to development*. Participation Group, Institute of Development Studies.
Giddens, A. (1982). From Marx to Nietzsche? Neo-conservatism, Foucault, and problems in contemporary political theory. In A. Giddens (Ed.), *Profiles and critiques in social theory* (pp. 215–230). Macmillan.
Hadot, P. (1995). *Philosophy as a way of life: Spiritual exercises from Socrates to Foucault*. Blackwell.
Halbwachs, M. (1995). Collective memory and historic memory. *Revista Española De Investigaciones Sociológicas, 2*(69), 209–219.
Halbwachs, M. (1996). Collective memory and time. *Cahiers Internationaux de Sociologie, 101*, 45–65. http://www.jstor.org/journal/cahintsoc
Hall, S. (1997). *Representation: Cultural representations and signifying practices*. Sage & Open University.

He, L., & van Heugten, K. (2020). Chinese migrant workers' care experiences: A model of the mediating roles of filial piety. *Qualitative Health Research, 30*(11), 1–13. https://doi.org/10.1177/1049732320925420

Hobsbawm, E. J., & Ranger, T. O. (1983). *The invention of tradition*. Cambridge University Press.

Hodder, R. (2000). *In China's image: Chinese self-perception in Western thought*. Macmillan.

Hook, D. (2001). Discourse, knowledge, materiality, history: Foucault and discourse analysis. *Theory & Psychology, 11*(4), 521–547. https://doi.org/10.1177/0959354301114006

Huang, J. (2011). *The reproduction of filial piety in a community: Discourse and practice*. Social Sciences Academic Press.

Jing, J. (1996). *The temple of memories: History, power and morality in a Chinese village*. Stanford University Press.

Kockelmans, J. J. (1972). *On Heidegger and language*. Northwestern University Press.

Ladany, L., Yan, S., & Zhang, W. W. (2013). Mazu Daoyi (Ma-tsu Tao-i). In *Encyclopedia of Chinese philosophy*. People's Press.

Lewis, D. (1983). New work for a theory of universals. *Australasian Journal of Philosophy, 61*(4), 343–377. https://doi.org/10.1080/00048408312341131

Lin, X. (2013). *Gender, modernity and male migrant workers in China: Becoming a 'modern' man*. Routledge.

Luo, C. (2013). *Filial piety and its "tianjingdiyi" 天经地义论孝道*. Guang Ming Ri Bao 光明日报出版社.

Luo, Y. (2011). Reading Halbwachs's 'the collective memory.' *Research on Northwestern Ethnicities, 2*(1), 87–101.

Manning, K. E., & Wemheuer, F. (2011). *Eating bitterness: New perspectives on China's Great Leap Forward and famine*. UBC Press.

May, T. (2006). *The philosophy of Foucault*. Acumen.

O'Farrell, C. (2007). Key concepts [webpage]. *Foucault News*. https://michel-foucault.com/key-concepts/

Oliver, P. (2010). *Foucault—The key ideas*. Teach Yourself.

Ouyang, Q. (2012). Foucault's new political perspective: A genealogical construction of micro-power. *Journal of Renmin University of China, 2*(2), 90–102. http://research.ruc.edu.cn/Article/ShowClass.asp?ClassID=24

Rosen, S. (2007). *Mao's last revolution*. Harvard University Press.

Shen, V. (2012). In search of modernity and beyond: Development of philosophy in the Republic of China in the last hundred years. *China Review International, 19*(2), 153–187. https://doi.org/10.1353/cri.2012.0033

Sheridan, A., & Foucault, M. (1980). *The will to truth*. Tavistock.

Smith, J. A. (2008). *Qualitative psychology: A practical guide to research methods* (Vol. 2). Sage.

Song, Z. (2008). *Chinese traditional philosophical discussion 中国传统哲学通*. People's University of China Press.
Song, Z. (2013). People's University of China: Heritage & Chinese traditional philosophical discussion '中国人民大学: 薪火传承&中国传统哲学通论'. YouTube: iCNTV中国公开课官方频道 China Public Class Official Channel.
Tu, W. (1976). *Neo-Confucian thought in action: Wang Yang-Ming's youth (1472–1509)*. University of California Press.
Tucker, M. E. (1991). The relevance of Chinese neo-Confucianism for the reverence of nature. *Environmental History Review, 15*(2), 55–69. https://doi.org/10.2307/3984970
Wang, C. (2016). Return to the ethical subject: Foucault and Confucian modern values 重回道德主体: 福柯与儒家现代价值. *Tianfuxinlun 天府新论* (3), 58–63. http://www.tianfuxinlun.com/ch/index.aspx
Wang, D. (2010). *The fall of humanity 人类的没落*. Xianxi People's Publisher.
Wang, D. (2016). The one with no fear has a heart of fear: Three fears of Junzi and its educational purpose for youth 无畏者怀有的敬畏之心——君子三畏及对青年的借鉴意义. *Social Science 社会科学:全文版* (12), 00047. http://www.cqvip.com/QK/72177X/
Willig, C. (2008). Discourse analysis. In J. A. Smith (Ed.), *Qualitative psychology: A practical guide to research methods* (Vol. 2). Sage
Xian, Z. (2013). Critique of Foucault's theory of discourse. *Theoretical Studies in Literature and Art, 1*(1), 121–129. http://tsla.ecnu.edu.cn/EN/volumn/current.shtml
Xu, Y. (2007). Death and dying in the Chinese culture: Implications for health care practice. *Home Health Care Management & Practice, 19*(5), 412–414. https://doi.org/10.1177/1084822307301306
Yan, Y. (2006). The pattern of difference classification and the Chinese cultural perspective on classification 差序格局与中国文化的等级观. *Social Science Research 社会学研究* (4), 201–213. http://www.shxyj.org/
Zhang, X. (2017). Mainland contemporary neo-Confucianists and neo-Kangyouweiism 大陆新儒家与新康有为主义的兴起. *Aspects of Cultural 文化纵横* (3), 98–107. http://www.21bcr.com/

CHAPTER 5

The Path to a Culturally Integrated Foucauldian Discourse Analysis

Introduction

My research aims to explore how participants perceive filial responsibility and the way they are influenced by external factors, such as culture, economic convenience, legislation, political propaganda, social insurance, and social norms, in carrying out their filial responsibility. Therefore, a social constructionist qualitative approach, which explores meanings in social context and people's subjective experiences, provides an appropriate fit. Both critical discourse analysis (CDA) and Foucauldian discourse analysis (FDA) are highly influenced by Foucault's theories on discourse and power. I arrived at the decision to employ FDA because of the flexibility of its methodological tools. FDA's flexible methodological positions come together with the subjective focus of my research questions, with the complexities encountered in the Chinese context, and with my attempt to develop a localised methodology. CDA provided a supplementary and complementary view on power inequalities experienced by migrant peasant workers and on gendered filial practices.

This chapter also links Foucauldian discourse analysis with Chinese philosophies in terms of their shared interest in action and practice and cultivation of the self. By connecting these two perspectives, they were able to build on the common grounds, thus enabling a localised approach to the research. In addition, this orientation ensures theory is relevant to understanding and potentially ameliorating (taking action in relation to)

L. He, *Care Work, Migrant Peasant Families and Discourse of Filial Piety in China*, https://doi.org/10.1007/978-981-16-1880-2_5

human problems, which is appropriate for a study located in the discipline of health sociology and other areas of social science.

In the latter half of this chapter, the research design and fieldwork procedures for this study are explained in detail. During fieldwork, I grew as an interviewer and as a researcher as I dealt with anticipated and unanticipated issues, such as trying not to anticipate the answers of participants. I reflected on my positionality which involved perspectives gained as both an insider (from the same hometown and speaking the same language) and an outsider (not a migrant peasant worker nor sharing care experiences for parents diagnosed with terminal cancer) to the dilemmas faced by my participants. The self-reflexivity I undertook during all stages of the research, including during the transcribing of interview recordings, equipped me to be more attentive to my participants' subjectivities and develop more professional research skills.

Research Questions and Objectives

This study aimed to examine the complex construction of filial piety in the context of end-of-life care. It further sought to discover how the socio-economic changes that followed on from economic reform interact with migrant peasant workers' experiences of fulfilling filial responsibilities. Primary sources of data were the accounts of end-of-life care experiences of migrant peasant workers in China who were looking after parents with terminal cancer. In exploring the research questions, my research objectives were to find out how the participants constructed their discourse and what this discursive construction might reveal; in what ways these constructions can be understood; how complex filial discourses are constructed through various contextual factors; and how power relations are mediated between and among governmental discourses and subjective discourses of filial piety, especially when different political agendas contradict one another.

Qualitative Research and Social Constructionist Underpinning

In the following sections, I explain my selection of qualitative methodological approaches and the social constructionist approach I adopted in my research.

Qualitative Research

This research investigated how migrant peasant workers made sense of filial piety through end-of-life care experiences. It endeavoured to understand how they perceived and conceptualised their care experiences. The ultimate goal was not principally to construct theories but to uncover the complexity of participants' narratives about filial perceptions and practices with (or without) forming certain theories. Therefore, a qualitative approach to research was deemed to be fitting for this endeavour.

Although the flexibility of qualitative research is generally considered to be a bonus, Morse (2012) criticised qualitative research for being too fluid; its flexibility can be abused. It is therefore also important to ensure qualitative research is appropriately grounded in cohesive methodological approaches that are consciously selected and reflected upon throughout the research.

Social Constructionist Underpinning

A social constructionist approach was used to uncover the ways in which participants experience caregiving while embedded in a context where discourses of filial piety shape familial and other important relationships (Burr, 2015, p. 2). Although in many qualitative research projects, constructionism and constructivism are used interchangeably without making any apologies for doing so (Lynch, 1998), in this research, social constructionism was chosen as I considered it to be a better fit. Without doubt, constructivist and constructionist perspectives have much in common (Lynch, 1998). Both of them claim that meanings and knowledge are created within a social context. However, social constructionism focuses on how meaning is created through shared production often among groups of people, while social constructivism focuses on how individuals make meaning through their interaction with social contexts (Young & Collin, 2004). Although my research drew on individual interviews its purpose was to theorise about the experiences of a social group, namely Chinese migrant peasant workers. Instead of focusing on individuals as autonomous beings who are engaged in identity construction and delving into subjective internalisations of participants, this research endeavoured to investigate knowledge construction that takes place within social contexts and through social actions.

Putting the difference between social constructivism and constructionism aside, it is important not to overlook that social constructionism can attend to micro-level considerations of how individuals construct themselves and each other through interaction (Burr, 2015, pp. 14–24). In theorising about my findings, my constructionist ontological position did not induce me to adopt an extreme structuralist position as opposed to an extreme agency position. For instance, in Chapter 7, internally constructed feelings such as fear, guilt, and gratitude are discussed. However, this research is more inclined towards the macro-level considerations of social construction. This macro-level position towards the analysis is in part influenced by, and reciprocally influences, my choice of FDA, which focuses on individuals' representation of social construction through deconstructing texts and other discursive sources (Burr, 2015, pp. 23–26), rather than discursive psychology, which focuses on individuals' internalisation of social construction (Burr, 2015, pp. 23–26).

Social constructionism deals with how various realities of individuals in a particular setting are socially constructed (Ritchie et al., 2013). Constructionist views of social phenomena examine the constructed understandings of a particular situation, specifically through an individual's interactions with the social world (Mills et al., 2006). It comes from a place where assumptions about discursive reality are shared by individuals and groups of individuals. It focuses on how human beings invent themes from the social world and share and make sense of these themes through texts, language, and discourse (Mills et al., 2006). My research centres on a shared Chinese cultural norm, that of filial piety. Filial practices, such as taking care of one's parents when they are old or sick, might not only exist in the Chinese context. However, the discursive realities that people construct to arrive at the meaning of filial piety may differ in different cultures. Thus, social constructionism invites a critical view of taken for granted realities/knowledge. At the same time, it realises that all understandings are culturally and historically relevant (Burr, 2015, pp. 3–4). One of the major criticisms of social constructionism is that the researcher's positioning might impose his/her cultural and historical specificity on participants (Burr, 2015, pp. 3–4). As a researcher who was born and raised in Langzhong, the place where this research was conducted, I realised that occasionally I tended to anticipate a particular answer even before I had asked participants a question during an interview. As a matter of fact, when I went back to listen to the interview recordings, I found that I sometimes repeatedly asked participants the same questions just to get the answer I wanted. Such taken for granted views were discussed with my supervisor through Skype meetings when I was in the field, and I tried to avoid these pitfalls in later interviews.

The epistemological nature of social constructionism demands a connection between researcher and participants (Lofland & Lofland, 1995). Such a connection is accepted as an inseparable element of locating and constructing knowledge in qualitative research. In this research, I am investigating filial perception and practice through participants' eyes, in my own interpretation. There is no absolute objective knowledge according to this approach. Qualitative researchers acknowledge the contextual influences on both researcher and participants (Lofland & Lofland, 1995). As a researcher, I needed to constantly reflect on my own position while interacting with my participants and the surrounding context. Doing this helped me to improve my interviewing skills and I became more nuanced in my approach. My position as a Chinese researcher who was born in the same city as my participants and also as someone who studied and worked in a faraway country away from my parents did not categorise me as a migrant peasant worker, but it did provide me with some shared experiences. Additionally, my caregiving experience for my mother, who was diagnosed with benign tumours during the research, also made me somewhat of an 'insider'. Still, I am not a migrant peasant worker, nor can I be considered socially marginalised. I might have some shared caregiving experiences with my participants, but my mother did not have terminal cancer.

Most of my tertiary education has been undertaken in western countries, which affected how I structured my interview questions and research design. As Gair (2012) stated, qualitative research has moved away from dichotomous and towards more fluid conceptualisations of insider and outsider status. Being familiar with the locality and language of my participants granted me constructive ways of understanding what they were trying to say to me. On the other hand, being aware that I was influenced by other perspectives, such as those that I had acquired through studies in western societies, helped me to adopt a position of 'uncertainty' and resist and question preconceived notions about similarities (Nowicka & Ryan, 2015, p. 1). The importance of nuanced understandings of positionality will be elaborated later.

Methodological Decisions

As discussed in Chapter 4, Hall (2001) explained Foucault's concept of discourse as follows:

> Discourse, Foucault argues, constructs the topic. It defines and produces the objects of our knowledge. It governs the way that a topic can be meaningfully talked about and reasoned about. It also influences how ideas are put into practice and used to regulate the conduct of others. (Hall, 2001, p. 72)

Discourse analysis refers to the observation of patterning of language as well as the circumstances such as situations, participants' social groups, purposes, and outcomes with which these patterns are characteristically associated socially, economically, culturally, and politically (Wodak & Meyer, 2009). Social constructionists emphasise that language is performative and provides a site for people constructing knowledge and meaning (Burr, 2015). Owing to consideration of the study of languages *in use* as a medium of social construction and change, discourse analysis is best suited to researchers who are seeking to integrate theories and practices (Wodak & Meyer, 2009). A social constructionist approach can employ various research tools such as discursive psychology, conversation analysis, Foucauldian discourse analysis, interpretative repertoires, narrative analysis, and CDA (Burr, 2015, pp. 170–202). FDA was decided on as my main methodology because it is an extremely useful approach for examining different social phenomena and for revealing how language is implicated in power relations.

Foucauldian Discourse Analysis and Critical Discourse Analysis

In my research, Foucauldian understandings revealed how conscious cultural perceptions of filial piety were shaped in a temporal and spatial context that was governed by interactions of power and discourse (van Dijk, 1993). The cultural perception of filial piety is something fluid, because it constantly constructs itself through people's various discourses, where change emerges in alignment with relevant social positionings. For Foucauldian discourse analysts, meanings of words and texts are fluid because they flow among various discourse constructions through processes such as subjective positioning (Hook, 2001). This fluidity enables change to happen (Hook, 2001). For FDA, discourse can be written texts, interview audio records, participatory observed actions, or anything else that carries meanings for FDA (Hook, 2001).

According to Burr (2015, pp. 190–192), FDA deals with two further questions or processes, other than just examining language in use by people. It also considers social structures and material conditions in which discourse takes place, and investigates practices implicated in particular discourses (Burr, 2015). Also various forms of discursive construction are interlinked. In the context of my research, this draws attention to how filial discourse is also closely linked with other discourses such as informal care discourse, discourse of the contemporary Chinese intergenerational relationship, neoliberal discourse, governmental political discourse, and so on. Moreover, discourse of filial piety can be both constraining and productive, as is emphasised in Foucauldian notions of power (Lin, 2013); FDA's complex approach to considering relational power dynamics considers that power is relational and operates in a web-like fashion. Therefore, FDA became my main methodological tool, although I borrowed some aspects of CDA as complimentary tools for raising questions about the data.

Like FDA, CDA often challenges the taken for granted assumptions in everyday discourse (Fairclough, 1993). Taken for granted ideologies construct a hegemony that Foucault called disciplinary power (Conradie, 2011). The inequalities faced by migrant peasant workers and the historically gendered nature of filial piety (e.g., the daughter-in-law used to carry out all the hands-on care for her husband's parents) led me to draw on CDA's methods for questioning social inequalities among marginalised social groups.

CDA often draws on news reports and government policy releases for analysis to criticise the discourses of institutional and public settings (Burr, 2015; Conradie, 2011). CDA focuses on the practical linking of political and social engagements (Wodak & Fairclough, 2004). I explored these links by considering some pertinent government documents and news reports in my research. Although CDA was not chosen to be the main methodological approach for my research, its take on social inequalities and resistance of taken for granted hegemonic discourses, especially its critique of institutional discourses, assisted in the data analysis. This research drew theoretical and methodological inspiration from literature on CDA.

The writing of important critical discourse analysts such as Wodak, Fairclough, and van Dijk helped further my understanding of Foucault, because they were deeply influenced by Foucault in theorising their own CDA methodological approaches. Critical discourse analysts developed numerous methodological instruments partially based on Foucault's theory (see Wodak's historical discourse approach, Fairclough's textually oriented discourse analysis, and van Dijk's socio-cognitive approach; van Dijk, 2009; Wodak & Fairclough, 2004; Wodak & Meyer, 2009). In my research, which involved an attempt to include Chinese philosophical tools to account for *Chineseness*, I arrived at a more flexible methodological foundation of FDA; Foucauldian discourse analysts often do not have a set methodological framework and instead analyse discourse through Foucault's key ideas (Hook, 2001).

Approaches to Foucauldian Discourse Analysis

Andersen (2003) identified three main stages for FDA, synthesising these from Foucault's writings. Firstly, archaeology was described by Foucault himself as an appropriate way to analyse local discursivities (Foucault, 1972). This is generally identified as the first stage of Foucault's work, which asks an essential question: why did this narrative occur, instead of another? (Andersen, 2003). Archaeology is neither a methodology nor a full-fledged theory but rather a critical and careful exploration of an object of study (Webb, 2012). According to Dreyfus and Rabinow (1982), Foucault was fully aware of the social constructionist nature of archaeology, no matter how hard he tried to avoid it. When a discourse occurs in a particular place, the influence of social institutions on the discourse is often discussed and presented in archaeology (Dreyfus & Rabinow, 1982).

The second stage of Foucault's discourse analysis is known as genealogy. It presents techniques for subjective knowledge to be used to assess contextual, networked, and historical operations of the discursive object, with a shift in theoretical focus to consider power relations (Andersen, 2003; Foucault, 1972). Genealogy was a method that Foucault resorted to once he found himself in a dilemma over fundamental assumptions about causal power within the structuralist approach (Steigmeier, 1998). Foucault's genealogy originated from Nietzsche's genealogy, which entailed the development of a method that would allow him to make up some 'random' connections that could unsettle the only perceived history (Dreyfus & Rabinow, 1982). Yet, for some Foucauldian scholars, genealogy starts from asking questions such as why the question should be asked (Hook, 2001). Hook gave up exploring the deep layer of linear history, since there is no generalised history of societal development (Hook, 2001). History is seen by some as only a repeating never-ending drama of the governance of power (Foucault, 1972). In my research, I follow Hook's rejection of deep analysis of linear history. However, 'random' connections are explored and found to dismantle the perceived history, as was recommended by Dreyfus and Rabinow (1982).

In Foucault's genealogical perspective, nothing is 'natural' or truthful; there is no perception of a certain and solid way of existence, but rather, existence is created and recreated in an ever-changing network of power and knowledge co-creations and interactions (Xu et al., 2020). Therefore, entrenched perceptions such as perceptions of what is 'natural' need to be examined archaeologically and genealogically.

Andersen (2003) emphasised genealogical analysis of institutional practice (governmental practice in my research) and how it interacts with the formation of filial discourse. According to Foucault (2000), power is everywhere, but not an entity that institutions (such as the government) or people can obtain and thereafter hold. As he explained,

> If one wants to analyze the genealogy of the subject in Western civilization, one must take into account not only techniques of domination but also techniques of the self. One must show the interaction between these types of technique. (Foucault, 1997, p. 177)

According to Bartelson (2001), Foucault depicted the immanent rational function that the state has and 'must' deploy to maintain a certain order. Foucault attempted to deal with the concept of the state and recognised

> that the existence of the state has been accepted as a point of departure by many scholars ... since all inquiry simply has to start from somewhere in order to get anywhere ... even those who have struggled hard to reconceptualize the state and political order have failed to escape statism themselves ... it is nevertheless held together by a common critical spirit that seems to gravitate towards the state just in order to breathe life into it through the unmasking gestures characteristic of that spirit. (Bartelson, 2001, pp. 27–28)

Other Foucauldian scholars, such as Sidhu (2003), also claimed that the exercise of institutional power is a very important form of power relations within any particular society.

In my research, the power relations between governmental discourse and filial discourse were explored to understand participants' discursive construction of filial piety in contemporary Chinese society. I followed Andersen's emphasis on the analysis of institutional practices by examining the practices of the Chinese government.

The first two stages, archaeology and genealogy, lead to the final stage of FDA, which is *care of the self*. This stage investigates the way individuals realise that they are discursive subjects (Andersen, 2003; Willig, 2001). In my research, this stage mainly focused on examining the participants' discourses in order to figure out how they constructed their subjective positions and filial self.

In my research, the question of how structure and agency relate is not explicitly and overtly discussed but instead is brought together by drawing upon two Foucauldian discourse analysts: Hubert L. Dreyfus and Paul Rabinow. They were two of the early Foucauldian scholars who comprehensively and coherently examined Foucault's work (Dreyfus & Rabinow, 1982; Frohmann, 1994). They believed that understanding the deepest meaning of a topic under investigation through its history is the only way for human science to proceed (Dreyfus & Rabinow, 1982). They claimed that it is possible to reconcile self-subjectification (agency) and a structuralist view of social science (structure) (Dreyfus & Rabinow, 1982). They claimed to have conceived a method, 'interpretive analytics', that describes Foucault's work and achieves such reconciliation (Dávila, 1993). Interpretive analytics advocates that archaeological and genealogical constructions are appropriate tools to study the history of thought (Dávila, 1993). Interpretive analytics is not used as a methodological tool in my research, but it does help build the theorising process of archaeological and genealogical analysis of my data. The balanced view of structure and agency applied in interpretive analytics is adopted in my research. As Dávila (1993) said, power, knowledge, and the self form the axes for experiences. In my research, both the idea of self-subjectification and structuralist views are presented and utilised.

Even though scholars such as Andersen, Dreyfus, and Rabinow all claimed that they developed an approach to FDA derived from Foucault's work, their methodology is not systematic. In particular, they have tended to neglect the importance of practice (in contrast to language). Another influential Foucauldian discourse analyst is Carla Willig. Her six steps of FDA (Willig, 2008) propose a relatively clear and cohesive approach that explicates the practice-oriented definition of discourse, which was an important consideration in my choice of approach. The six stages to perform FDA, according to Willig (2008), are discursive constructions (themes/foci of discourses), discourses, action orientation (indicators of personal stances on statements about discourse), positioning (subjects within the structure of rights and responsibilities), practice (ways through which discursive constructions react to opportunities for action), and subjectivity (feelings and thoughts experienced) (Smith-Merry, 2014; Willig, 2001, 2008).

Owing to the structured (and step-by-step) approach to analysis, many scholars, especially research students, tend to adopt her framework as their methodological tool because they think the steps help to simplify FDA. However, even when the six steps are closely examined, it becomes clear that the connections between her six steps remain complex and multidirectional (Smith, 2008); simply providing a name for each step does not make analysis any easier or more systematic (Smith, 2008). Nonetheless, Willig's emphasis on practice and action orientation provided helpful clarifications for my research. Firstly, her focus on action orientation demonstrates that practice is also a form of discourse. According to Foucault, discourse is not just language, but also actions and practice (Foucault, 1970). In a sense, discourse connects everything and includes everything. Secondly, Willig's work shed light on how participants constructed discourses to make sense of their filial practices and actions, and consequently reconstructed their practices and actions through those constructed discourses.

Chinese Epistemological Positioning

Chineseness. Before I delve into Chinese epistemological considerations and how these relate to FDA, I will first briefly define Chineseness for my research. In his book *Peasant Society and Culture: An Anthropological Approach to Civilization,* Redfield (1956) claimed that there are two types of tradition: *great tradition* and *little tradition*. Great tradition refers to the culture represented by thinkers and scholars; it is seen to involve philosophising through deep and reflective thoughts. Little tradition refers to the everyday life of people, especially the more marginalised groups, such as migrant peasant workers in my research. These two dimensions of traditions interact with and influence each other. According to Li (1996), great tradition focuses on philosophical thoughts and sophisticated language, while little tradition starts from everyday needs, and is thereby practical and straightforward. He thought that while it is important to undertake research into the philosophy and belief systems of a particular culture, people's everyday lives and practices could be an even stronger reflection of the core foundation of Chinese culture and tradition.

According to Huang (2011), the differentiation of the two kinds of traditions is often vague and overlapping in the Chinese context. Great tradition can be considered to relate to the approach to education and governing taken by the Chinese empire in ancient times. But she argued that, in Chinese culture, the relationality discussed in Chapter 4, makes it difficult to differentiate the two forms of traditions. Filial piety is associated with both forms of tradition. On the one hand, filial piety is a foundational aspect of Confucianism, as well as other ancient Chinese philosophies (He & van Heugten, 2020). On the other hand, filial piety has been integral to long-term social practices of Chinese people for thousands of years.

A quality of unease or unsettledness can be discerned in relation to the idea of Chineseness in current Chinese society. In the last century, as mentioned in Chapter 2 and Chapter 3, Chinese philosophy was forcefully or willingly replaced by western philosophies and theories associated with western modernity. However, people's everyday life still embodies thousands of years of tradition and cultural practices (Huang, 2011). Thus, there is an unsettling imbalance between western theories and Chinese people's everyday life. Chineseness, therefore, refers to people's everyday life and practices that are still in association with Chinese traditional philosophies and thoughts.

Action-orientedness. Four years into this research, I encountered my own epistemological dilemma. Wittgenstein used the term 'language game' to explain how the meaning of language changes in different contexts (cited in Kopytko, 2007). If I might borrow this term to describe my own struggles, I became frustrated by 'language games'; I reflected on how many social scientists appear to be obsessed with the vocabulary that they and others employ to explain or interpret certain points of view. The focus seemed to be overwhelmingly on understanding and expressing meanings instead of on being action-oriented. I could not help but wonder about the debate between the social sciences and hard sciences, and whether there is some merit in the idea that social science is not scientifically valid and not particularly useful, as might be proposed by hard scientists and by others who might critique its frequent lack of action-orientedness.

According to Harari (2014) in his book *Sapiens: A Brief History of Humankind,* human history unfolds in close relationship with non-socially constructed variables such as biology and geography. Foucault's thinking in the last years of his life suggested that people have the ability to change their subjective positioning (agency). However, this agency is limited if everything is socially constructed (Burr, 2015). In my estimation, structure partially depends on the 'generic traits' of objects. Social structure is not limitlessly dependent on imaginations and perceptions. For example, the terminal cancer faced by my participants' parents resulted in a very limited life expectancy. My participants wished their parents could live many more years but they knew this was not possible. In other words, while social constructionism appears to reject the existence of reality outside socially constructed knowledge (Parker, 1998), perhaps not everything is socially constructed, and I began to wonder how helpful a constructionist position was to people like my participants. This dilemma became one of my major struggles.

It was not until I started to search for a relationship and points of connection between discourse analysis, to be precise FDA, and Chinese philosophical underpinnings that I finally arrived at some kind of resolution. Similar to the way in which Chinese philosophies always put a focus on actions/practices, Foucault also talked about the further implication of actions through subjective positioning within a particular discourse. Such action perceptions do not focus on a never-ending struggle between objectivity and subjectivity and how this is bounded by a certain perceived reality but rather are more inclined to 'act' in order to make a change or possibility happen. This impelled me to continue my research, carrying my epistemological confusion along rather than becoming frozen by my inability to resolve this. As Elder-Vass (2012) stated, some social constructionists are critical realists who do not deny the connection between knowledge and objects, even though they reject that there is a knowable objective reality and truth outside of social construction.

As discussed in Chapter 4, many Chinese philosophers valued action more than philosophical inquiries into the nature of knowledge. Chinese philosophy both transcended and participated in human activities and social interactions (Song, 2008). There were philosophers such as Laozi (ca. 604–ca. 531 BCE) who spoke about Dao (道, the way), which created the universe, and how people should practise and choose actions according to 'the way' (Feng, 1995). There were also philosophers such as Confucius (551–479 BCE) who taught ethical and behavioural virtues and regulations to ordinary people (Feng, 1995). Confucius once said that studying the *Book of Poems* is a prerequisite for governing (Song, 2008). Zen Buddhism also valued the way of *rushi* 入世—practising Buddhism in a worldly, engaged way, as opposed to by withdrawal from society and by seeking solitary spiritual cultivation—and engaging with human society and social issues (Song, 2008). The famous Zen Master Mazu Daoyi (709–788) said that the way of becoming a Buddha is not through reading and chanting Buddhist books and meditating but through *rushi* and practising Buddhism (Ladany et al., 2013). According to Zhou et al. (2016) and Cheng (2009), for the philosophies discussed above, the most important element of filial piety was that it is by nature pragmatic. Cheng (2009) argued that the valuing of the action/practice of filial piety infiltrates into every aspect of Chinese people's everyday lives, through discourses of filial piety.

This philosophical view of knowledge/action was also embodied in my participants' narratives. Many participants felt reluctant to tell their parents they loved them or to use the word love when speaking with the interviewer. As a Chinese person myself, I have also never literally said 'I love you' to my parents. However, this does not mean that Chinese people do not express love for their parents. One enables parents to know one's love by carrying out actions that show this love or care. In my research, participants came back to take care of their ill parents and provide full or at least partial financial assistance to cover all their expenses. To the participants, these actions are much more important than simply saying 'I love you'. Wang Fuzi's dialectic underpinning of knowledge and action is seen here. Zhong and He (2014) suggested that there is a fundamental western bias towards seeing 'self-disclosure and verbal expression' as the key forms of interpersonal intimacy and as the appropriate focus of discourse analysis. Instead, they suggested, more concrete actions and actual interpersonal collaborations may better define a discourse about intimacy and individuation within the filial piety relationship. It was therefore essential for me to attend to this broader conceptualisation of discourse in my research, and both FDA and Chinese philosophical perspectives helped me to do that. This ensured, for example, that I took notice of participants' practical expressions of caring in my fieldwork observations.

For Foucault also, language and discourse were performative and action-oriented (Burr, 2015). Foucault furthered his theoretical explorations by examining the implications of actions in particular discourses (Burr, 2015). Discourse generates knowledge and also implicates actions and practices. Many ancient Chinese philosophies did not specifically discuss the origins of knowledge. Wang Fuzi (1619–1692) claimed that knowledge came from action and practice (Liu, 2004). This action/practice approach to knowledge and values that is embedded in Chineseness has been able to reach a consensus with Foucault's discourse theory, as Foucault also valued action and practice as an essential part of discourse (Foucault, 1978; Zhang, 2015).

The action/practice philosophical tradition is still embedded in Chinese scholarship today. For example, contemporary Chinese philosopher Shen (2012) re-examined Confucius' thought and developed the Confucian idea of *shu* (altruistic extension), recommending an action/practice of going beyond oneself to embrace many others. This action/practice goes beyond the relational self of Confucius' ideology, and counters postmodern relativism (Shen, 2012). Shen (2012, p. 181) claimed that 'one should draw one's own ideas and values out from one's world [Chineseness] and then put them into other people's world [western modernity] to see whether they are valid there'. His theory may not be sufficiently comprehensive, but it provides a starting point for the negotiation of the unsettling relationship between Chineseness and westernisation.

Cultivation of the Self. Another struggle I had at about the same time during my research journey related to a question about culture. To what extent should a social science researcher need to define the scope of the concept of culture? When a social phenomenon is investigated in relation to a certain culture, what moral positioning is appropriate as a health sociologist, in terms of viewing the possibility of change for that social phenomenon? For example, if participants do not tell their parents that they are terminally ill, should I fully accept this 'cultural' practice, or might I think that another approach could be more beneficial for the parents/patients? As a social science researcher, it is ethical to leave judgement about 'good' and 'bad' (e.g., about whether a participant is a good filial son or a bad one) out of my analysis. However, when and to what extent is it appropriate to move forward and analyse the concept, possibilities, and benefits of change? Another similarity between Foucault and Confucianism (earlier identified in Chapter 4) enlightened me on this. The technique of self-cultivation helped me to consolidate or at least move forward, carrying along with me the contradictions within current discourses on cultural issues.

Foucault's explanation of parrhesia can be summarised as follows:

> Parrhesia is a kind of verbal activity where the speaker has a specific relation to truth through frankness, a certain relationship to his own life through danger, a certain type of relation to himself or other people through criticism … and a specific relation to moral law through freedom and duty. More precisely, parrhesia is a verbal activity in which a speaker expresses his personal relationship to truth, and risks his life because he recognizes truth-telling as a duty to improve or help other people (as well as himself). In *parrhesia*, the speaker uses his freedom and chooses frankness instead of persuasion, truth instead of falsehood or silence, the risk of death instead of life and security, criticism instead of flattery, and moral duty instead of self-interest and moral apathy. (Foucault, 1999, p. 5)

Confucianist tradition similarly regards 'self-cultivation as the foundation of a personhood, and also his lifelong duty' (Kai, 2008, p. 22). Ivanhoe (2000) identified that the Confucian tradition of *self-cultivation* contains a duty of telling the truth. Heubel (2008) tried to develop a cross-cultural methodology for modern Chinese issues, starting from the common ground between Foucault and Chinese philosophies (mainly Confucianism) on cultivation of the self. Irrespective of criticism about the fundamental differences between Foucauldian and Confucian self-cultivation, the notion of parrhesia provides encouragement to social researchers to frankly tell the 'truth' out of sincerity and a strong sense of duty, especially in uncomfortable scenarios (Mackie, 2007). Some of the 'truths' I arrived at in my research, the critiques I developed, were uncomfortable to express because although I undertook my research at a western university, I am Chinese and careful in steering a course between facile criticism of, for example, Chinese governmental policy and avoidance of making such criticisms for (quite possibly unnecessary but nevertheless real) fear of negative repercussions befalling me.

Summary of Methodological Foundations. The considerations outlined in the above discussion further solidified my conclusion that FDA was the most appropriate methodological approach for examining the narratives of the participants for this particular investigation. My supervisors and I exhaustively discussed the logic of using a methodology based on western philosophy to investigate a 'purely' Chinese construct. Ultimately, and recognising that Chinese and western philosophies have already inevitably encountered and engaged with one another for over a century in the Chinese context, we determined that it was appropriate to adopt an approach that can reflect both theoretical foundations. This also recognised that with the rejection of traditional thought and philosophies during Mao's era (and even before that), it has become very challenging for Chinese scholars to adopt a completely 'Chinese' methodological view to do 'scientific' research, even in the social sciences.

Most Chinese scholars understand Chinese philosophies at least partially through the eyes of western hermeneutics (Liu, 2004). This might seem like a rather pessimistic view of Chinese philosophy. However, as reflected in Foucault's thoughts on hegemony, subjective positioning of agency allows changes that can resist hegemonic discourses. Moreover, there is no doubt that current Chinese society has been 'modernised' to a great extent. The study of Chinese culture and values, such as filial piety, through FDA, can contribute to both Chinese and western literature. The scientific bias that Eastern philosophy is unscientific, emotional, and subjective limits the ways in which the study of Chinese culture can be explored, and this study aims to contribute to an understanding of how the limitations of 'localising' a western or more precisely a (post)modern theory on an aspect of Chinese culture can be overcomed.

Foucault was highly critical of modernity and modern scientific disciplines and endeavoured to seek solutions in the far past (Feng, 1995; Song, 2008). Perhaps it is meaningful to look back into ancient Chinese philosophy, just as Foucault did when searching for possible solutions in ancient Greek and Roman history (Foucault, 2005, 2012; Zhang, 2015). Ultimately, FDA provided me with some guidelines and parameters within which filial piety could be examined that allowed for both flexibility and robustness in the analysis of data. Along with the complementarity of CDA and relevant Chinese philosophical thought, this research adopted its own unique 'mixed' methodology.

Research Design

Following the start of my PhD studies (in January 2013), my research proposal had been rewritten several times owing to shifts in my research objectives and my understanding of research design. An example of an interesting and influential event that happened occurred at the end of my proposal stage. The Chinese government enacted the 'Parents Visiting Law' (Elderly Rights Law), which became effective from 1 July 2013. I realised that I could now explore the otherwise potentially difficult to approach topic of how governmental discourse affected participants' filial perception by asking questions about this new law. Policy documents in relation to this (and other laws) were identified as another important source of data.

The next important step required before embarking on fieldwork involved applying for ethics approval from the University of Canterbury Human Ethics Committee. Important strategies indicated in the application included measures to protect participants' identities through the use of pseudonyms and the secure storage of all raw data. The seeking of approval is only a first step in undertaking ethical research; ethical issues that emerged will be discussed later in this chapter.

As discussed earlier in this chapter, this research is qualitative. The main data was obtained through semi-structured interviews. After the proposal stage and before I went back to China to undertake fieldwork, I created questions and guidelines for the interviews and discussed these with my supervisor. We agreed that the scope of questions and guidelines was sufficient for data collection. The day I returned to my hometown, which was also my research field, I found out my mother was ill and hospitalised (the same hospital as my main designated participant recruitment site). I took care of her in the hospital for almost two months before I started my interview phase. This very personal experience gave me clarity on how to approach my potential participants with sensitive questions (e.g., questions related to their parents' approaching death). I also gained perspective on how to approach potential participants in the hospital setting. For example, family members of patients were required to spend long periods of time at the hospital to take care of their ill parents. After they got used to my presence in the hospital they were more likely to talk to me and share their stories. In the next few sections, I will talk about the research design and process in more detail.

Participant Inclusion Criteria

There is no consensus about the number of participants that should be interviewed in FDA research (Bidet, 2010). Too few might hinder the researcher from collecting enough useful data for the research; too many would present an impossibly large task to accomplish for a doctoral project. The methods involved in-depth, open-ended interviews and a questionnaire right after the interview. After discussion with my research supervisors, I estimated that 20–40 participants needed to be recruited for this research. The inclusion criteria for participants were, first, that they must be the sons, daughters, and/or daughters-in-law of people living with advanced cancer, where patients could be expected to survive for at least a few months after professional diagnosis. The participants needed to have worked in a city remote from their home village at least at some stage of their lives (so that they identified themselves as *minggong* or migrant peasant workers). Sons-in-law do not traditionally engage in filial caregiving activities in China and thus were not included as potential participants in this study. Patients with cancer were also not participants in this study; the participants were the adult children of such patients. Because not all adult children engage in visible forms of caregiving and would define themselves by the term 'caregiver', this term was not used in recruiting participants. Instead, sons and daughters, as well as daughters-in-law, were included in the recruitment regardless of the way they defined themselves in relation to this situation.

All of the participants in the study were migrant peasant workers, a group that represents the majority of workers in rural China. Migrant peasant workers were selected as study participants as they represented the more 'traditional' concept of filial piety. The participants were the primary caregivers, and it was expected that their narratives would characterise how filial piety is practised in a rural setting. Notably, caring for their terminally ill parents required the participants to stay with their parents and be unemployed for the period they had to provide this care. The participants' caregiving activities therefore determined their use of time, and often meant they needed to change their location, moving to centres where their parents were hospitalised.

Site Selection

The study was conducted in a small city called Langzhong in the large province of Sichuan in China, wherein there has been a marked increase in the incidence of cancer among its citizens.

Sichuan is the second largest labour export province in China. It has a low level of GDP per capita (Xu et al., 2019). In 2010, 13.6 million people were below the poverty line, which made Sichuan the second poorest province in China (Xu et al., 2019). Sichuan has a population of 81 million people in the year 2018; 15 million of these are migrant peasant workers who go to other provinces to work and live (Xu et al., 2019).

Langzhong is a county in the north-eastern economic zone of Sichuan. Langzhong has a population of approximately 840,000, one-third of whom are registered as rural residents of Langzhong (Xu et al., 2018). As mentioned in Chapter 2, the incidence of cancer in China has doubled in the last decade, and cancer has become the leading cause of mortality in rural China (Xu et al., 2018). 'Cancer village' is a term that has become increasingly employed in both the Chinese and western media to describe places with high rates of cancer. As a likely result of water and other pollution associated with industrial development, stomach, liver, and oesophageal cancer rates appear to be much higher than the world average in China. According to Liu (2010), Sichuan has been reported to contain four 'cancer villages' in governmental documents. However, according to Lora-Wainwright, there may be a lot more of these villages as the incidence of cancer still tends to be underreported. Langzhong has been recognised as one of the regions with very high rates of cancer in China, especially for oesophageal cancer. Most of the patients in the cancer centre where the present study was conducted had oesophageal cancer; the rest had stomach cancer. Thus Langzhong was chosen as the research field because of the likelihood of successful recruitment of enough participants. Moreover, the research setting provided the rural context that was important in this research. Finally, Langzhong is my hometown and this location therefore offered practical and financial as well as academic advantages.

Recruitment

Two recruitment methods were adopted in the field: convenience sampling and snowballing (both word-of-mouth, acquaintance-based processes). The majority of recruitments took place in the biggest local hospital, Langzhong People's Hospital. With the assistance of the director of the cancer centre, the criteria for sampling were refined to facilitate the selection of suitable potential participants.

I was in the hospital most afternoons for four–five months when the field research was being carried out. The recruitment and interviews usually took place in the afternoons because potential participants were heavily occupied in the morning: because participants were often the main caregivers in the hospital, they needed to constantly monitor the intravenous drip [or: feeding tube] and other machines, wait for the doctors' daily rounds, and attend to other chores. In every patient's room were potential participants who met the inclusion criteria, according to the information provided by the director. However, in discussion with the research centre, it was agreed that the best way to approach the potential participants was when they were physically far from their parents. This was to ensure that patients (who were not research participants) would remain unaware of the interviews or the research study (children might not want their parents to know about the cancer). This sampling was mainly based on convenience. In the end, 20 participants agreed to participate and 19 completed both the interview and questionnaire data collection parts.

Because some cancer patients might not be able to afford treatment at a hospital or decide not to go through treatment for other reasons, I also drew on the assistance of an acquaintance to develop and post an advertisement on a notice board in a central part of Langzhong city (this approach had received prior approval from the University of Canterbury Ethics Committee). This approach did not attract additional participants. A snowballing approach did result in five additional participants being introduced to me through my extended family and an acquaintance. Therefore, a total of 24 interviewees participated in the study. Because one of the participants was working in a remote city at the time of the interviews, a telephone interview was conducted with that participant. After the 24th interview and after reviewing the interview notes, the decision was made that sufficient data had been collected, and I decided not to recruit any more participants.

Care had been taken to ensure that confidentiality was protected and clearly explained in informed consent forms. I also ensured there were provisions for necessary assistance such as free counselling or debriefing sessions for the participants, should these be required. The recruitment and interviewing process took approximately three to four months (between the end of 2013 and the beginning of 2014), and I was required to follow strict guidelines set by the cancer centre's director, such as not to disturb patients who required rest and not to disclose information to the patients without permission. Interviews were recorded and transcribed, and permission was sought from the participants for this recording.

Data Collection Methods

Interviews

The main data-gathering method used in the study consisted of semi-structured interviews with the recruited participants. According to He and van Heugten (2020), in-depth interviews allow participants to use their own language to spontaneously and openly respond to questions. This facilitates a better understanding of people's perceptions (Punch, 2005).

The interviews were scheduled to fit in with participants' schedules and were conducted within the cancer centre. I used an interview guideline with open-ended questions that allowed flexibility and at the same time ensured that vital questions would not be left out during the interview. Interviews were free-flowing and the participants were encouraged to share their thoughts and feelings. An interview included four phases of questions: introductory questions, care task-related questions, questions about filial piety including spirituality, and questions about the new parent-visiting law and governmental and other support provisions and services. Each interview lasted between 1 and 3 h.

Survey Questionnaire

According to Dew (2007), there are no perfect approaches or methods for qualitative research, only suitable ones. By the time I undertook my analysis, I had grounded my approach in FDA and Chinese philosophies, with some consideration of CDA's concerns with inequality and gender; my approach to data collection included typical qualitative methods such as interviews, observation, and the sourcing of relevant documents.

A survey questionnaire was also used in the study. This survey contained questions about the demographic information of the participants as well as behaviours associated with caregiving. The questionnaire asked about age, relationship to the patient, number of children, number of dependents, number of siblings, marital status, employment, monthly income, living expenses, financial support, and perception of the filial self.

There were also open-ended questions in the survey questionnaire; these aimed to elicit descriptions of the realities of filial being and the filial self.

Although in the proposal stage the survey questionnaire was planned as a convenient way to collect supplementary demographic data and other quantifiable information, such as how many hours it takes to travel to the hospital, the research quickly evolved to adopt a more constructionist focus. With hindsight, the survey could have been avoided had I appreciated a constructionist approach more fully from the outset. Nevertheless, its inclusion probably assisted some participants who appreciated its concrete approach. The data did provide some illuminating details, and rather than either ignoring the survey results (and potentially disrespecting the participants' efforts to respond) or presenting these to quantify information and support a hypothesis, in Chapter 6, personal information is used to provide a background for participants' stories and comments about their experiences.

Observation and Field Notes

This study also employed the use of naturalistic observations; the participants in the study were observed during their daily interactions in the cancer centre in which the study was conducted. On days when I was unable to recruit any participants, I offered to assist participants in caring for their parents and to be a companion to the participants and the patients. Conversations needed to be discretely managed in the presence of the patients in particular because, as is the norm in China, patients invariably had not been advised of their diagnosis by their doctors or their families. Some participants did not feel comfortable accepting my offer (as was expressed by them) and then the offer was set aside; some expressed gratitude. Some useful narratives were obtained after the interview when I was able to interact with the participants in an informal setting such as in the smoking area. Observations enriched my data and enabled me to consider the context in which discourses were formed and constrained.

I wrote field notes to document the observations made each day as well as the key occurrences that were observed in the field. These field notes contextualised the interview data and supported my identification of themes that emerged in the research data.

Policy Documents and News Reports

Relevant documents on filial legislation and policies from different historical stages of Chinese society were examined. Documents were obtained using University of Canterbury library search engines, Google Scholar, Wangfang search engine, Zhongguo Zhiwang search engines, and Baidu scholars. These documents were examined to complement the discourse analysis of collected data from the field and revealed further information about current discourses on filial piety.

Ethics and Informed Consent

With the help of the director of the cancer centre, prior to any interviews, I provided potential participants with information letters and consent forms and briefly explained the content and benefits of this research. The letter contained general information about the research and its purpose. The concept of confidentiality was explained to potential participants and they were informed that after the interview's conclusion they would receive a supermarket coupon worth NZ $10 (¥ 47.96) or gifts of similar value such as milk, biscuits, or other gifts patients usually receive in the hospital as a token of gratitude. They were informed that they could withdraw from the research at any point. Ethics approval was also obtained from the hospital authorities (including service staff and doctors) to ensure staff would not feel that the boundaries of their workspace were infringed without their consent.

Further verbal explanations were provided at the start of interviews, including about the topic of the research and what types of questions would be asked. Participants were again reassured that their answers would be kept confidential. Given the situational context, wherein participants were dealing with a terminal illness affecting their mother, father, or parent-in-law, emotions were likely to be heightened, and discussing this situation in the interviews was expected to potentially generate distress. To address these concerns, a local therapist who specialised in stress and grief was consulted about the research. His advice regarding how to deal with the potential distress of the participants in the context of local culture was sought before any interviews were conducted.

Although it was expected that grief, stress, and sorrow might manifest during the interview process, it also seemed likely that participants might benefit from the opportunity to talk about their experiences and to reflect on things they did not usually reveal to other people. Fortunately, no participants wanted to end the interview because of emotional distress, even though they were told that they could withdraw at any moment if they did not feel comfortable. During the interviews, I found that participants were not as outwardly distressed or as emotional as I had expected them to be. This may be a function of culture since most Chinese children have been trained to control their emotions from a very young age. Provisions were made in case participants might need professional help in managing their emotions. The local therapist whom I had consulted before my fieldwork was made available to the participants free of charge, and they were informed that if they experienced difficulty in dealing with their emotions following the interview, I would help them to access therapy sessions. Although a number of participants asked for the therapist's name and contact number, none of the participants contacted the therapist during the fieldwork.

In the research design, the potential issue of discovering elder abuse while in the field was considered due to increasing rates of elder abuse in recent years in China (Dong et al., 2007). The possibility created a significant ethical dilemma for me. Certainly it would be helpful to collect information on elder abuse as it would provide an honest and truthful account of what is happening in today's families. However, if I did not report the incident to the authorities, it would be unethical; yet at the same time, reporting to authorities would violate the confidentiality agreement made to participants. The Chinese law that forbids elder abuse does not provide comprehensive criteria for the identification of elder abuse, particularly emotional abuse (Dong et al., 2007). People still widely accept the traditional perspective that elder abuse is simply a family matter (Nie, 2019). Chinese authorities tend to avoid using criminal standards to deal with elder abuse-related matters, even though there is a criminal law forbidding such activities; instead, they often apply persuasion and make referrals to family counselling (Dong et al., 2007). Moreover, older persons rarely report abuse to the authorities owing to the cultural importance of saving face—it would be intensely shaming to admit to being abused by one's child—and fear of losing family support (Dong et al., 2007). Ethical standards concerning research with human participants specifically state that the researcher should guard against any undue harm to participants; elder abuse is a different story, however. Elder abuse can pose a serious threat to the life and well-being of the patient, and in discussion with my supervisors prior to entering the field, I determined that I would have a moral obligation to alert the authorities to this matter. I did not warn participants that if I identified abuse I would need to report it since this might deter them from participating in the study. In the end, I was relieved that no elder abuse was identified in the field.

I stood in a unique position in terms of interviewing the affected individuals because, as a fellow native of Langzhong who had also cared for a parent in that hospital, the participants were willing to talk to me. For fear of causing trouble for friends and colleagues, participants often did not share their dilemmas in relation to filial responsibility; as some participants explained, telling colleagues or friends about a parent's illness might be perceived as a subtle demand for money or gifts.

Anticipated and Unanticipated Issues

Initially, some difficulties were encountered in recruiting participants. Firstly, timing was one of the key aspects to determining whether a potential participant would be willing to take part in the research. Potential participants were often too busy to spare any time in the morning, because this is when they were heavily engaged in caring for their ill relative. The first four potential participants withdrew from the research within the first week due to this reason. Secondly, many people in China feel reluctant to be interviewed, especially about political issues, and especially when they know they are being recorded (Heimer & Thøgersen, 2006). The interview was designed to ask participants' opinions about a range of relevant matters including governmental policies and formal and informal support, and there were several potential participants who refused to participate mainly due to the fact that the interviews were going to be recorded. A relative mistrust of social science research was also likely to be involved. According to Liu (2010) there is an association between modernisation and an increasing scam rate in Chinese society. The more a society is 'modernised', the higher the rate for scams in that society (Liu, 2005). Criminals tend to use social research as a way to obtain people's personal information in order to defraud them of their money and other assets (Liu, 2010). This may explain why some potential participants frowned when they were approached. Furthermore, talking about death is still perceived as taboo in China, especially a parent's impending death (Sayer, 2010). This taboo subject was bound to be discussed in these interviews.

During the interview stage, several issues emerged. Firstly, some participants had trouble answering questions while dealing with their strong emotions during the interview. According to Foucault (1972), researchers commonly encounter obstacles to obtain detailed information from participants due to social, cultural, and familial pressure, or for fear of losing face, especially with a stranger. Some of my participants would try to avoid discussing issues such as how to take care of dying parents in detail. I always paused and gave them time to decide how to proceed. If they showed signs of distress or discomfort, I asked them whether they would like to stop the interview. None of the participants wanted to stop the interview because of emotional distress. Instead, several went on to emphasise their responses through repetition, which, although indirectly, showed their strength of feeling about their parents' illness, and indicated that they valued the opportunity to speak about this in confidence.

Secondly, there is a presumption that Chinese people are afraid to speak about the government since this may result in government or police intervention. This idea is not only widespread among western people, but also among Chinese people including myself. However, in recent years the Chinese government has opened up many sensitive areas for researchers, including in relation to health, welfare, and justice, and criticism about the government's policies has become more possible (Bakken, 2000). As anticipated, some participants were not comfortable to criticise governmental policies. However, there were others who were not afraid to talk about the government's performance in a critical manner.

Thirdly, in the interview design, I had intended to explore the spirituality of participants. While a spiritual discourse can be identified within participants' narratives in response to certain questions, participants found it difficult to understand the questions directly pertaining to the topic. As someone who is Chinese, it is extremely difficult to translate the idea of spirituality. The difficulty does not involve matters of linguistic translation. Chinese people were forced to abandon religious beliefs during the Cultural Revolution. Moreover, people were manipulated to only believe in communist materialism. Spiritualties were seen as unimportant and as a luxury of capitalism. Therefore, it was almost impossible to explain spirituality to participants. Due to the demographic group chosen in this study, oftentimes they had not received much formal education, and there was a need to use plain language to communicate.

In contemporary Chinese society, spirituality is often considered as something more pertaining to the white-collar class or as a privilege enjoyed by wealthy people (Zhong, 2017). This is in stark contrast with how spirituality is considered in western literature on the end-of-life, as well as among laypeople in western communities (Atchley, 2009; Murdock, 2005; Tacey, 2004). In China, people who practise or identify with spirituality might be assumed to be rich (or middle class), well-educated, and liberal. In this way, spirituality became something I presumed the participants might not understand due to their social status, and because I presumed it to be a western concept to which they might not have had access. Yet at the same time, in much of the western end-of-life care literature, caregivers are said to gain comfort from spirituality, and spirituality is considered to help them deal with their care burdens (Colgrove et al., 2007; Kaye & Robinson, 1994). However, none of the participants understood what spirituality meant during the interviews. The Chinese word I found to be closest to spirituality is *jingshen* (精神, non-material/inner strength and spirit). And perhaps, in part due to also being Chinese, I struggled with the concept myself.

Gender Issue

Gender has been a subject of interest in filial piety research, and it has been noted, for example, that in traditional China the eldest daughter-in-law was the main source of instrumental care for aged parents. The increasing need for urban workers has led to expectations that women will join the urban workforce, and this has also contributed to changes in filial practices. The norm regulating filial practices, according to which an eldest son's wife should live with, and care for, her parents-in-law, is weakening, according to Chen (2009). In traditional China, a daughter-in-law would stay at home under the authority and supervision of her parents-in-law, while men went out and engaged in economic activities (Cong & Silverstein, 2008; Loong-Yu & Shan, 2007).

Since Mao's period, women have been encouraged to go out and find work (McDaniel & Zimmer, 2013). Since the economic reform, there has been a great need for a female workforce from rural areas in the mass production industries (Cong & Silverstein, 2008). According to Yan (2003), in 1993, the number of rural women migrant workers had reached 263,000, which accounted for nearly 40% of the migrant workforce. Through their employment, rural daughters have acquired new social roles, gained some economic independence, and increased their economic value to their parents (Cong & Silverstein, 2008). The care-giving pattern has been significantly altered by this change (Cohen & Deliens, 2012). Owing to the one-child policy, parents invest in sons' and daughters' futures equally, which is a marked change from historical practices (Yu, 2018). The wife of the eldest son no longer has to stay at home and provide full-time care to her parents-in-law. She will tend to care more for her own parents, who have invested in her as they would in a son (Hooyman & Kiyak, 2008). Koshy (2013) argued that daughters are more concerned with their own parents, partially owing to the 'debt-bound value' that ethical morality complies with (whereby children repay the sacrifices made by their parents). The literature about these topics is largely descriptive, however, and gender analysis is often missing.

Research done by Deutsch (2006) to compare university graduates from one-child families with those with siblings and to investigate filial piety and patrilineality found that the only child (no matter if male or female) felt especially responsible for their parents' health and happiness. Deutsch (2006) also found that among both one-child families and those with siblings, patriarchal belief is evidently weak. Another scholar, Lee (2012), undertook research among one-child families and those with siblings about gender equality in education, and discovered that gender equality was significantly enhanced among one-child families in terms of education. In my research, the gendered nature of filial piety is considered, although only to the limited extent that it emerged as relevant to the data. To more deeply investigate this topic would require further study (see in Chapter 10).

Positionality: Beyond Insider and Outsider Dualities

Due to my anticipation of difficulties in recruitment, I had asked the director of the cancer treatment centre to assist me during the recruitment process. However, it turned out there were many people willing to be interviewed without his help. This may have been due to the fact that, like the participants, I was from a rural area near the city of Langzhong. Thus, participants may have expected that I would be familiar with how Chinese culture and filial care (including any burdens) were perceived by them. This familiarity likely helped participants to open up during the interviews. Dwyer and Buckle (2009), in reflection of their own studies, asserted that qualitative researchers are often faced with dilemmas about maintaining the 'space between' insider–outsider positions in qualitative research. While sometimes researchers are left with little option but to respectfully acknowledge, as relative outsiders, the experiences shared by participants, as relative insiders, many researchers are not clearly either insiders or outsiders. In this research, because the research took place in my hometown, I might be considered an insider researcher. Although no 'cultural' ambiguity was anticipated, an insider might easily take things for granted and miss important information. For example, some information relating to local/general conditions was already known to me. Due to this, I sometimes persisted in asking participants a question repeatedly until the expected answer was obtained based on my preconception of reality. Fortunately I spotted this early on in listening to recordings of initial interviews.

Additionally, no matter how hard I tried not to impose moral judgements on participants, my presumed knowledge about local/general realities continued to interfere with my attunement to participants during interviews. For example, one participant said, 'I communicate with my heart. They [my siblings] only provide whatever my father needs materially'. He was saying that he paid more attention to the emotional needs of his father compared to his siblings. He believed that his emotional care was considered more important by his father, compared to his siblings' financial care. To me, it sounded like the participant was not doing his best to be filial because he did not provide enough financial assistance. In this context, people are often looked down upon when they do not provide financial assistance to their ill parents, especially if they are sons. I was influenced by that common judgement. My judgement was further fuelled when some participants explicitly asked me to help them settle some matter or other with the government.

However, later in the analysis, I reflected on Dreyfus and Rabinow's introduction to an interview with Foucault that 'once one sees the pervasiveness, dispersion, intricacy, contingency, and layering of our social practices, one also sees that any attempt to sum up what is going on is bound to be a potentially dangerous distortion' (Dreyfus & Rabinow, 1982, p. xxv). To generalise on the basis of so-called underlying truths of perceived cultural construction will generate distortions (Steigmeier, 1998). Thus, my understanding of my own culture might have created a distorted moralistic judgement of some participants. Such judgements inevitably occur during a discursive analytical process; when their biased nature was noted, this also led to a better understanding of discourse analysis. After all deficit discourse is as important as other discourses. The analysis became a process of reflexivity, and also raises an inquiry about the dilemma Foucault did not resolve. That is, he focused on the relationship of power and discourse to avoid dealing with questions of morality and value generated from dominant discourses (Dreyfus & Rabinow, 1982). However, value and morality are mainly created within hegemonic discourses in Foucault's depiction of discourse (McMahon, 2000).

While I was doing my analysis and writing my thesis, my mother was diagnosed with numerous new tumours in her digestive and reproductive system. It took me a few months to take care of her and I remained with her through the time of her surgeries. Although my fieldwork was by now completed, I began identifying with my participants, for example when I was filled with fear that my mother too might have cancer and die. As a result of my anxiety, I resumed smoking after having quit a long time before. This experience, and the fact that I am Chinese, provided me with an insider's perspective on my research topic. However, I needed to be careful with my presumptions. As previously noted, most researchers are both insiders and outsiders; insider and outsider positions are not binary. For instance, my mother was not 'dying', and I am not a migrant peasant worker. I was still also an outsider. Moreover, adopting a western theoretical basis also meant I retained an outsider view to an extent. For Geertz, it is important to embrace a different culture from a humble position and an acknowledgement of one's outsider point of view (Geertz, 1994; Inglis, 2000). This requires researchers to listen carefully to what participants are trying to say, by attempting to stand in their shoes. I accepted I was both an insider and outsider and tried to avoid the detrimental impacts that result from either position. To sum up my experiences within the domain of the insider–outsider non-dichotomous position, owing to the relation-oriented nature of Chinese culture, my identity became a subject of constant negotiation and renegotiation through interaction with the participants. Eventually, this prolonged interaction with the participants allowed my reflexive position to evolve and enabled me to appreciate the importance of uncertainty (Nowicka & Ryan, 2015).

Self-Reflexivity During Data Collection Procedures

The concepts of filial piety and migrant peasant workers' subjective experiences of their filial selves are abstract and difficult to define. Data collection was designed to obtain participants' discourses derived from filial care experiences.

The interview itself provided a social context both for participants and for me. Helping a participant understand a certain question presented a difficult task on some occasions. Breaking down an academic concept into simple language requires strong communication skills and relevant life experiences, as well as knowledge of related cultural settings. I made progress over time, especially after acquiring lay language from the participants to help me to better explain my questions.

I began to realise that I was often unconsciously judging participants' competency and capacity to understand and mistakenly presuming these to be lacking. For example, I tried to use much easier and non-technical or lay language to initiate questions to older participants, due to the intergenerational difference in public education levels. However, it turned out that most of the older participants did not have any difficulties understanding me and even taught me many idioms. At the same time as providing appropriate guidance, I also needed to take care to not overly influence or lead participants' responses. On the other hand, some participants also appeared to be influenced by their preconceptions about my identity. For instance, older participants appeared to believe they needed to present a role model (including in relation to filial practices) to me—the younger researcher.

The first participant in my research, after the formal interview was completed, scolded me for not teaching her how to answer my questions prior to the recorded interview. This, she asserted, would have enabled her to give 'better' answers. I had to explain to her that the interview was not a journalistic interview and the transcript would not be read as such by other people.

Just as participants tried to give 'better' answers, however, I also wanted to provide better explanations for questions. The interview recordings were always reviewed in the same evening, in order to reflect on interview skills and question design for future interviews. It was very uncomfortable to listen to my interviewing style. I was disappointed in my interviewing skills, a feeling that persisted right up until the end of the fieldwork. However, it was a necessary process for me to learn.

As an interviewer, the main task is to elicit and prompt narrative accounts from participants. When some participants felt threatened or feared losing face during the interview because they worried that in their answers they might not match the interviewer's intelligence, I explained that I was not the expert and that the participants were the experts. Even though this mindset could not be completely altered, notable shifts in openness could be seen following these explanations, and responses became more narrative-based instead of being constituted by answers such as 'I am not well educated, I do not know how to answer this one'. When participants felt nervous about the recording procedure, I explained to them that this was 'not an interview but a conversation'. When there were silences and pauses during interviews, I learned not to force the participants to respond because this was likely to lead to participants providing information to merely satisfy the interviewer. Instead, participants were prompted to further explain their ideas. When the conversation touched on topics that might accrue social stigma, I tried to be as non-judgemental as possible. For example, some participants might not be able to provide hands-on care for their ill parents. If I had asked questions such as 'Do you provide hands-on care to your parent?' participants would have been likely to evade the question and not provide a frank answer. Instead, I asked, 'How do you provide support for your parents when you are not physically present?' This appeared more likely to elicit uncensored responses.

The interviews were conducted in Chinese, and hence there was an initial issue with translating or using the right words to convey what had been said in the interviews. The interview recordings were transcribed word for word in Chinese prior to being translated into English. One of my supervisors, who is a native Chinese speaker, checked my translations. My other supervisor also gave helpful comments on some English expressions I had mistranslated.

Data Analysis

As mentioned above, several Foucauldian scholars' analytic ideas and frameworks are partially adopted as tools for this research, such as Andersen's (2003) three steps for analysis. Archaeology provides the descriptive explanation of how knowledge is managed (Diaz-Bone, 2003). It examines the emergence of a discourse through describing the evolution of the smallest statements (Andersen, 2003). It contains more formal knowledge such as that obtained from books and archives and other forms of institutional knowledge (McKenzie & Scheurich, 2008). Genealogy focuses on power, knowledge, and their relationship (Vakirtzi & Bayliss, 2013). It examines the wider social, historical, political, and cultural context of a particular discourse, and involves a search for different realities that are presented in that discourse (Andersen, 2003). The literature review investigated past research, governmental archives, and other formal documents and this formed the basis for archaeological research and a genealogical examination of the discourse of filial piety. As discussed before, it is almost impossible to separate these two forms of analysis. Therefore, in practice no particular division between these two forms of analysis was drawn. The data was also examined using the third phase of the methodology: care of the self. This phase involved exploring how participants' subjective position within the context of the archaeological and genealogical aspects was determined and how it affected their construction of the filial self.

Hook's (2001) thoughts on rejecting deep analysis of history as it is disruptive were adopted to complement the genealogical analysis of the historical path of filial piety. 'Random connections' of sudden breaking points in history were explored in accordance with Dreyfus and Rabinow (1982), in particular in relation to the impacts of the New Culture Movement and the Cultural Revolution. Discourse analysis led to the examination of previous literature and documents relating to the practice of filial piety and how it has been transformed through the influence of culture, politics, and economics. The impact of this approach to analysis can already be seen in the literature review chapter. The 'care of the self' method enabled the examination of how participants' subjective position was determined within the context of the archaeological and genealogical aspect, and how this subjective position affected their construction of the filial self. This approach to analysis was complemented by Willig's (2001) focus on practice and actions. When discourse generates knowledge, power, and the subjective self, it also derives from these at the same time. In the same manner, discourse is (re)constructed through, as well as (re)constructive of, practice and action. Particularly, how participants' practices and actions shaped their discursive formation of filial burden, filial responsibility, the filial self, and governmental discourse was examined using Willig's (2001) ideas on these two steps.

Although the analysis of the data adopted FDA methodology and methods, the present research was guided by the richness of the data and the different themes that emerged from its subjective content. Instead of letting the methods guide the data analysis, I tended to find similarities between themes as they arose, and employed relevant methods that included FDA, Chinese metaphysics and theories, and, to a lesser extent, CDA. Thus, the analysed narratives were more interpretative and reflective. For example, the participants' narratives revealed what is 'doable', 'thinkable', or 'sayable' and accepted in a specific time and place. Their narratives changed and at times appeared contradictory, for example in both praising and criticising governmental policies in care of the dying, and in both disagreeing and agreeing to tell their parents about cancer. The public identities of the participating 'children' as obedient filial subjects were discovered to be partially produced by a discourse that was mainly focused on the identification of the history of parental sacrifices that require reciprocation through end-of-life care by their children. Discourse analysis was used to reflexively and critically investigate participants' stories in order to question the power relations of formed discourses (parents, children, and the government) and how such discourses marginalise children of the dying and achieve children's construction as sole caregivers. This questioning of perceived ideas makes possible the idea of change, wherein new relations and practices in filial piety might occur.

FDA is also used in exploring migrant peasant workers' construction of the filial self. To understand the variable discourses on one object through different subjects provided a way to resist dominant discourse. It is crucial to attempt to understand the deep meanings of participants' narratives, and thereby to identify various discourses as opposed to solely focusing on dominant discourses. For Foucault, to deny the existence of deep meaning was to neutralise discursive variety and heterogeneity (Hook, 2001; Wickham et al., 2005). From an FDA perspective it is also essential to recognise and attempt to understand multiple social realities in a particular cultural setting. This is important in relation to my research topic, since children's relationships with parents vary in different socio-historical contexts (Wickham et al., 2005). It is important always to bear in mind that deep meaning was one of the objects of study for Foucault (Hook, 2001). In keeping with that aim, this research has been grounded in reflective analysis (Steigmeier, 1998).

Conclusion

In order to explore how filial piety is constituted and considered, this study used a qualitative approach, specifically discourse analysis, as its research methodology. A qualitative approach allowed me the flexibility to interact with my participants and data. Furthermore, a constructionist and discursive view was applied as the epistemological underpinning for the qualitative method. A constructionist qualitative approach deals with reflection on constructed realities of individuals in certain social, political, cultural, and economic circumstances, through their language, discourse, and practices (Gergen, 1996). Discourse analysis evolved from such perspectives and allows researchers to examine the way knowledge is created within various discourses and their interconnectivities (Gergen, 1996; van Dijk, 1993). In my research, within the discursive approach, underlying paradigms of FDA (and some CDA literature resources) were utilised to understand the narratives of participants in their relevant social contexts. While FDA led me to examine the position of power in the hands of dominant governing institutions in the society (the Chinese government in this research), it also shed light on less unidirectional power relations and the complexity of various discourses participants constructed around filial piety. A Chinese methodological underpinning, specially its focus on action and practice, was also used to complement the main methodology. This embedded this research within a Chinese cultural context and enables a possible bridge between 'Chineseness' and hegemonic western social science. FDA intrinsically challenges the taken for granted ideological power in the hegemonic system. Thus, taken together, this combination made an interesting mix of methodological tools and created a flexibility that was suitable for this research. Using such analytic tools, the next chapter will discuss participants' care responsibilities and burdens.

References

Andersen, N. A. (2003). *Discursive analytical strategies: Understanding Foucault, Koselleck, Laclau, Luhmann*. Policy Press.

Atchley, R. C. (2009). *Spirituality and aging*. Johns Hopkins University Press.

Bakken, B. (2000). *The exemplary society: Human improvement, social control, and the dangers of modernity in China*. Oxford University Press.

Bartelson, J. (2001). *The critique of the state*. Cambridge University Press.

Bidet, J. (2010). Foucault and liberalism: Rationality, revolution, resistance. *Critical Horizons, 8*(1), 78–95. https://doi.org/10.1558/crit.v8i1.78

Burr, V. (2015). *Social constructionism* (3rd ed.). Palgrave Macmillan.

Chen, S. (2009). Aging with Chinese characteristics: A public policy perspective. *Ageing International, 34*(3), 172–188. https://doi.org/10.1007/s12126-009-9043-6

Cheng, S. (2009). A discussion of the practicality of filial culture 简论孝文化的实践性. *Hubei University of Vocational Technology Publisher 湖北职业技术学院学报, 12*(4), 107–107. http://xb.wtc.edu.cn/

Cohen, J., & Deliens, L. (2012). *A public health perspective on end-of-life care*. Oxford University Press.

Colgrove, L. A., Kim, Y., & Thompson, N. (2007). The effect of spirituality and gender on the quality of life of spousal caregivers of cancer survivors. *Annals of Behavioral Medicine, 33*(1), 90–98. https://doi.org/10.1207/s15324796abm3301_10

Cong, Z., & Silverstein, M. (2008). Intergenerational support and depression among elders in rural China: Do daughters-in-law matter? *Journal of Marriage and Family, 70*(3), 599–612. https://doi.org/10.1111/j.1741-3737.2008.00508.x

Conradie, M. (2011). Masculine sexuality: A critical discourse analysis of FHM. *Southern African Linguistics and Applied Language Studies, 29*(2), 167–185. https://doi.org/10.2989/16073614.2011.633364

Dávila, J. (1993). Foucault's interpretive analytics of power. *Systems Practice, 6*(4), 383–405. https://doi.org/10.1007/BF01061958

Deutsch, F. M. (2006). Filial piety, patrilineality, and China's one-child policy. *Journal of Family Issues, 27*(3), 366–389. https://doi.org/10.1177/0192513X05283097

Dew, K. (2007). A health researcher's guide to qualitative methodologies. *Australian and New Zealand Journal of Public Health, 31*(5), 433–437. https://onlinelibrary.wiley.com/journal/17536405

Diaz-Bone, R. (2003). Developments in the field of the Foucauldian discourse analysis. *Forum Qualitative Sozialforschung/Forum: Qualitative Social Research, 4*(3). https://doi.org/10.17169/fqs-4.3.683

Dong, X., Simon, M. A., & Gorbien, M. (2007). Elder abuse and neglect in an urban Chinese population. *Journal of Elder Abuse & Neglect, 19*(3–4), 79–96. https://doi.org/10.1300/J084v19n03_05

Dreyfus, H. L., & Rabinow, P. (1982). *Michel Foucault: Beyond structuralism and hermeneutics*. University of Chicago Press.

Dwyer, S. C., & Buckle, J. L. (2009). The space between: On being an insider-outsider in qualitative research. *International Journal of Qualitative Methods, 8*, 54–63. https://doi.org/10.1177/160940690900800105

Elder-Vass, D. (2012). Towards a realist social constructionism. *Sociologia—Problemas e Práticas, 70*, 5–24. https://doi.org/10.7458/SPP2012701208
Fairclough, N. (1993). Critical discourse analysis and the marketization of public discourse: The universities. *Discourse & Society, 4*(2), 133–168. https://doi.org/10.1177/0957926593004002002
Feng, Y. (1995). *History of Chinese philosophy中国哲学史*. Zhonghua Shuju.
Foucault, M. (1970). *The archaeology of knowledge*. Tavistock.
Foucault, M. (1972). The confession of the flesh. In C. Gordon (Ed.), *Power/knowledge: Selected interviews and other writings 1972–1977* (pp. 194–228). Pantheon.
Foucault, M. (1978). *The history of sexuality (1st US ed.)*. Pantheon.
Foucault, M. (1997). *Ethics: Subjectivity and truth*, P. Rabinow (Ed.), R. Hurley (Trans.). The New Press.
Foucault, M. (1999). *Discourse and truth: The problematization of parrhesia; Six lectures given by Michel Foucault at the University of California at Berkeley, October–November 1983*. https://foucault.info/parrhesia/
Foucault, M. (2000). *The subject and power*. In J. D. Faubion (Ed.). The New Press.
Foucault, M. (2005). *The hermeneutics of the subject: Lectures at the Collège de France 1981–1982*, G. Burchell, Trans. Picador.
Foucault, M. (2012). *The history of sexuality (vol. 2): The use of pleasure*. Vintage.
Frohmann, B. (1994). Discourse analysis as a research method in library and information science. *Library & Information Science Research, 16*(2), 119–138. https://doi.org/10.1016/0740-8188(94)90004-3
Gair, S. (2012). Feeling their stories: Contemplating empathy, insider/outsider positionings, and enriching qualitative research. *Qualitative Health Research, 22*(1), 134–143. https://doi.org/10.1177/1049732311420580
Geertz, C. (1994). *Thick description: Towards an interpretive theory of culture*. Basic Books.
Gergen, K. J. (1996). Social psychology as social construction: The emerging vision. In C. McGarty, & A. Haslam (Eds.), *The message of social psychology: Perspectives on mind in society*. Blackwell.
Hall, S. (2001). Foucault: Power, knowledge and discourse. In M. Wetherell, S. Taylor, & S. Yates (Eds.), *Discourse theory and practice: A reader* (pp. 72–81). SAGE.
Harari, Y. N. (2014). *Sapiens: A brief history of humankind*. Harvill Secker.
He, L., & van Heugten, K. (2020). Chinese migrant workers' care experiences: A model of the mediating roles of filial piety. *Qualitative Health Research, 30*(11), 1–13. https://doi.org/10.1177/1049732320925420
Heimer, M., & Thøgersen, S. (2006). *Doing fieldwork in China*. University of Hawai'i Press.

Heubel, F. (2008). Cross-cultural critique and contemporary Chinese language philosophy: A reflection on the methodology of researching the late Michel Foucault 跨文化批判与当代汉语哲学—晚期福柯研究的方法论反思. *Scholarly Research 学术研究* (3), 5–13. http://mall.cnki.net/magazine/magalist/XSYJ.htm

Hook, D. (2001). Discourse, knowledge, materiality, history: Foucault and discourse analysis. *Theory & Psychology, 11*(4), 521–547. https://doi.org/10.1177/0959354301114006

Hooyman, N. R., & Kiyak, H. A. (2008). Opportunities and challenges of informal caregiving. In N. R. Hooyman & H. A. Kiyak (Eds.), *Social gerontology: A multidisciplinary perspective* (pp. 385–428). Allyn & Bacon.

Huang, J. (2011). *The reproduction of filial piety in a community: Discourse and practice*. Social Sciences Academic Press.

Inglis, F. (2000). *Clifford Geertz: Culture, custom, and ethics*. Polity.

Ivanhoe, P. J. (2000). *Confucian moral self cultivation*. Hackett.

Kai, D. (2008). Confucians' self-cultivation. *Journal of Jingmen Technical College, 8*, 22–29. http://www.en.cnki.com.cn

Kaye, J., & Robinson, K. M. (1994). Spirituality among caregivers. *The Journal of Nursing Scholarship, 26*(3), 218–221. https://doi.org/10.1111/j.1547-5069.1994.tb00317.x

Kopytko, R. (2007). Philosophy and pragmatics: A language-game with Ludwig Wittgenstein. *Journal of Pragmatics, 39*(5), 792–812. https://doi.org/10.1016/j.pragma.2006.04.011

Koshy, S. (2013). Neoliberal family matters. *American Literary History, 25*(2), 344–380. https://doi.org/10.1093/alh/ajt006

Ladany, L., Yan, S., & Zhang, W. W. (2013). Mazu Daoyi (Ma-tsu Tao-i). In *Encyclopedia of Chinese Philosophy*. People's Press.

Lee, M. (2012). The one-child policy and gender equality in education in China: Evidence from household data. *Journal of Family and Economic Issues, 33*(1), 41–52. https://doi.org/10.1007/s10834-011-9277-9

Li, Y. (1996). *Visual perspective of humanity 人类的视野*: Shanghai Arts 上海文艺出版社..

Lin, X. (2013). *Gender, modernity and male migrant workers in China: Becoming a 'modern' man*. Routledge.

Liu, J. (2005). Crime patterns during the market transition in China. *The British Journal of Criminology, 45*(5), 613–633. https://doi.org/10.1093/bjc/azi044

Liu, L. (2004). The Chuanshan theory's evolution, difficulty, and future 百年船山学的变迁、困境与出路. *Nantong Normal University Publisher: Social Science Edition 南通师范学院学报:哲学社会科学版, 20*(1), 149–153. http://www.21ks.net/shkx/shkx_15628.html

Liu, L. (2010). *Made in China: Cancer villages*. Taylor & Francis.

Lofland, J., & Lofland, L. (1995). *Analyzing social settings: A guide to qualitative observation and analysis*. Wadsworth.

Loong-Yu, A., & Shan, N. (2007). Chinese women migrants and the social apartheid. *Development, 50*(3), 76–82. https://doi.org/10.1057/palgrave.development.1100408

Lynch, M. (1998). *Towards a constructivist genealogy of social constructivism*. SAGE.

Mackie, P. F. E. (2007). Your philosophy of social work: Developing a personal and professional definition to guide thought and practice. *Journal of Social Work Values and Ethics, 4*(1), 1–20. http://jswve.org/

McDaniel, S., & Zimmer, Z. (2013). *Global ageing in the 21st Century: Challenges, opportunities and implications*. Ashgate.

McKenzie, K., & Scheurich, J. (2008). Teacher resistance to improvement of schools with diverse students. *International Journal of Leadership in Education, 11*(2), 117–133. https://doi.org/10.1080/13603120801950122

McMahon, C. (2000). Discourse and morality. *Ethics, 110*(3), 514–536. https://doi.org/10.1086/233322

Mills, J., Bonner, A., & Francis, K. (2006). Adopting a constructivist approach to grounded theory: Implications for research design. *International Journal of Nursing Practice, 12*(1), 8–13. https://doi.org/10.1111/j.1440-172X.2006.00543.x

Morse, J. M. (2012). *Qualitative health research: Creating a new discipline*. Left Coast.

Murdock, V. (2005). Spirituality and aging in the Bachelor of Social Work curriculum: Infusion and elective methods. *The Journal of Baccalaureate Social Work, 11*, 38–54.

Nie, Y. (2019). *The current status and affecting factors of elder abuse in China 中国老年人受虐待现状及其影响因素研究*. Doctoral dissertation, Jinan University.

Nowicka, M., & Ryan, L. (2015). Beyond insiders and outsiders in migration research: Rejecting a priori commonalities. *Forum Qualitative Sozialforschung, 16*(2), Art. 18. https://doi.org/10.17169/fqs-16.2.2342

Parker, I. (1998). *Social constructionism, discourse, and realism* (1st ed.). SAGE.

Punch, K. (2005). *Introduction to social research: Quantitative and qualitative approaches* (2nd ed.). SAGE.

Redfield, R. (1956). *Peasant society and culture: An anthropological approach to civilization*. University of Chicago Press.

Ritchie, J., Lewis, J., Nicholls, C. M., & Ormston, R. (2013). *Qualitative research practice: A guide for social science students and researchers*. SAGE.

Sayer, D. (2010). Who's afraid of the dead? Archaeology, modernity and the death taboo. *World Archaeology, 42*(3), 481–491. https://doi.org/10.1080/00438243.2010.498665

Shen, V. (2012). In search of modernity and beyond: Development of philosophy in the Republic of China in the last hundred years. *China Review International, 19*(2), 153–187. https://doi.org/10.1353/cri.2012.0033

Sidhu, R. K. (2003). *Selling futures: Globalisation and international education*. Doctoral dissertation, University of Queensland.

Smith, J. A. (2008). *Qualitative psychology: A practical guide to research methods* (vol. 2). SAGE.

Smith-Merry, J. (2014). Understanding talk and texts: Discourse analysis for nursing research. In M. De Chesnay (Ed.), *Nursing research using data analysis: Qualitative designs and methods in nursing*. Springer.

Song, Z. (2008). *Chinese traditional philosophical discussion 中国传统哲学通*. People's University of China Press.

Steigmeier, C. (1998). *Men in a cultural vise: Foucauldian genealogical analysis of the social construction of men as resistant*. Doctoral dissertation, University of Canterbury.

Tacey, D. J. (2004). *The spirituality revolution: The emergence of contemporary spirituality*. Routledge.

Vakirtzi, E., & Bayliss, P. (2013). Towards a Foucauldian methodology in the study of autism: Issues of archaeology, genealogy, and subjectification. *Journal of Philosophy of Education, 47*(3), 364–378. https://doi.org/10.1111/1467-9752.12004

van Dijk, T. A. (1993). Principles of critical discourse analysis. *Discourse & Society, 4*(2), 249–283. https://doi.org/10.1177/0957926593004002006

van Dijk, T. A. (2009). Critical discourse studies: A sociocognitive approach. In R. Wodak, & M. Meyer (Eds.), *Methods of Critical Discourse Analysis* (pp. 62–86). SAGE.

Webb, D. (2012). *Foucault's archaeology*. Columbia University.

Wickham, G., Potter, J., Willig, C., Hook, D., & Kendall, G. (2005). Commentaries on Hook, 'Genealogy, discourse, effective history: Foucault and the work of critique.' *Qualitative Research in Psychology, 2*(1), 32–46. https://doi.org/10.1191/1478088705qp026cm

Willig, C. (2001). *Introducing qualitative research in psychology: Adventures in theory and method*. Open University Press.

Willig, C. (2008). Discourse analysis. In J. A. Smith (Ed.), *Qualitative psychology: A practical guide to research methods* (vol. 2). SAGE.

Wodak, R., & Fairclough, N. (2004). *Critical discourse analysis*. SAGE.

Wodak, R., & Meyer, M. (2009). *Methods for critical discourse analysis*. SAGE.

Xu, D., Cao, S., Shui, Y., Liu, S., & Wang, X. (2019). The influence of social capital on location choice of migrant peasant workers: An empirical study in Sichuan 社会资本对农民工就业区位选择的影响——来自四川省的实证. *China Agricultural Resources and Division中国农业资源与区划, 040*(007), 66–73.

Xu, H., Wu, X., & Fu, L. (2018). An investigation of death caused by cancer among Langzhong residents from the year of 2011 to 2015 2011–2015年阆中市户籍居民恶性肿瘤死亡情况分析. *Journal of Preventative Medicine and Information预防医学情报杂志, 1*, 94–96.

Xu, J., He, L., & Chen, H. (2020). Balancing instrumental rationality with value rationality: Towards avoiding the pitfalls of the productivist ageing policy in the EU and the UK. *European Journal of Ageing, 17*(2), 251–257. https://doi.org/10.1007/s10433-019-00527-9

Yan, H. (2003). Specialization of the rural: Reinterpreting the labor mobility of rural young women in post-Mao China. *American Ethnologist, 30*(4), 578–596. https://doi.org/10.1525/ae.2003.30.4.57

Young, R. A., & Collin, A. (2004). Introduction: Constructivism and social constructionism in the career field. *Journal of Vocational Behavior, 64*(3), 373–388. https://doi.org/10.1016/j.jvb.2003.12.005

Yu, Q. (2018). *Has one-child policy positive influence on education level: Adopting RDD as a method计划生育政策提高了独生子女的受教育水平吗?--基于断点回归(RDD)的研究*. Doctoral dissertation, Wuhan University.

Zhang, X. (2015). An essay on Foucault's shift towards ethics in his late stage 论福柯晚期思想的伦理转向. *World Philosophy 世界哲学, 3*, 011. http://www.sjzxzz.cn/

Zhong, X., & He, S. (2014). Negotiating intimate relationships: Family relationship and filial piety expectations of parents of only children 协商式亲密关系: 独生子女父母对家庭关系和孝道的期待. *Open Times 开放时代, 1*(008), 155–175. http://www.opentimes.cn/

Zhong, Y. (2017). An exploration of stratification and social governing浅析中国的社会分层与社会治理. *Medium-and-small Enterprise Management and Technology (Mid) 中小企业管理与科技(中旬刊)*, (11), 102–103.

Zhou, S., Zhang, L., & Lan, X. (2016). Research review of filial culture in recent years 近年来孝道文化研究综述. *Changjiang Congkang 长江丛刊* (17), 36–37. http://128.qikan.qwfbw.com/

CHAPTER 6

Findings: The Burden of Care for Migrant Peasant Workers and Filial Piety's Mediating Roles

Introduction

In order to understand participants' subjective construction of caring for their parents at end-of-life and how these experiences related to discourses of filial piety, it is relevant to look at not only what care tasks participants took on but more importantly what impact these care experiences had on them. This chapter centres on participants' accounts of the challenges (including burdens) they encountered while providing care for their terminally ill parents.

According to Dreyfus and Rabinow (1982), Foucault's discourse theory rejects the idea that there is an underlying objective truth but instead 'seeks the surfaces of events, small details, minor shifts, and subtle contours' (p. 106). My participants expressed they had to face various challenges when caring for their parents with advanced cancer. Without trying to determine 'what is really being said or what may *not* have been said' (Steigmeier, 1998, p. 62), I focused on what it meant for care responsibilities or burdens to emerge in the participants' statements. I considered what happens when care challenges are constructed as either responsibilities or burdens. I drew on Foucault's reflections on madness wherein he emphasised that nothing exists outside of discourse (Foucault, 1967) to note that it is discursive formation that constructs meanings such as responsibilities and burdens. Although on the surface some of the content of participants' quotes could seem trivial and overly detailed,

L. He, *Care Work, Migrant Peasant Families and Discourse of Filial Piety in China*, https://doi.org/10.1007/978-981-16-1880-2_6

when read carefully these can 'provide the key to what is really going on' (Dreyfus & Rabinow, 1982, p. 102).

Foucauldian discourse theory encouraged me to bear in mind that discourses are by nature complex. Participants' filial discourses demonstrated that they constructed caregiving challenges neither solely as responsibilities nor solely as burdens. In fact, the interweaving of these two meaningful constructions showed how filial piety could simultaneously provide spiritual and cultural resources for taking on care responsibilities and become a hindrance to asking for help from outside sources to ease experiential burdens.

Different Forms of Care Impacts

All of the participants identified as migrant peasant workers (a direct translation of *nong min gong*) at least at one stage of their life. Their parents had resided in the rural area around the city of Langzhong for their whole lives whereas the participants had gone to the big cities for work. Analysis of the participants' responses to interview questions led to the identification of impacts of caregiving. There are several kinds of care impacts that are particularly burdensome for migrant workers, categorised as the emotional and physical impact of care, its financial impact, its work-related impact, and unfinished care and its impact. Additionally, gendered norms appeared to influence the form caregiving took and the impacts of caregiving on caregivers.

Emotional and Physical Impact of Care

Taking care of someone ill who is closely related can take a toll on caregivers, both emotionally and physically. Emotional and physical impacts are often interrelated. One participant described the emotional stress and physical burden she experienced while looking after her terminally ill father:

> When he is not around, the pain and fear of losing him is almost unbearable. I often cry with my mom in his absence. I feel like I have lost the ability to appreciate delicious meals. Sleep has become an issue for me since his diagnosis. ... I feel dizzy sometimes too. (P1: a daughter, aged 41–50, remarried, father was ill)

Financial Impact of Care

As migrant workers, most of my participants talked about the financial impact the parent's cancer had had on them. The son quoted below explained how expensive it was for migrant workers to come back to visit their ill parents. The second participant quoted below explained that as a migrant worker he could not afford all the expenses generated by his mother's illness, even if health insurance might cover some of these.

> All of my siblings are [migrant workers], so I had to make sure the diagnosis was right before I called them. If it was a small issue, it would cost a fortune for them to travel back. (P20: a son, aged 41–50, married, mother was ill)

> Money is an issue for such a major disease. Money doesn't fall from the sky, especially for peasant workers... We know there is medical insurance. However, we don't know how much it will cover. It might cover some [of the expenses], but who could help for the rest, and who would? It's [inadequate] for such a major disease. It will cost tens of thousands of RMB [Chinese dollars] for her disease, which I cannot afford. (P4: a son, aged 31–40, mother was ill)

The following statement further illustrated the disadvantaged financial position of migrant workers in the big cities and highlighted discriminatory practices that in many other countries would be illegal:

> You see, there is a lot of discrimination against us who came from interior China. We earn much lower wages than the local people do. (P15: a son, aged 41–50, married, mother was ill)

Work-Related Impact

The lack of proximity between migrant workers and their parents made care difficult to carry out, as demonstrated in this statement:

> In order to come back to see him [her ill father], I need to take a four-hour intercity coach to Guangzhou [the capital city of Guangdong Province] and then another 35-hour interprovincial coach to come back. I have a quite weak stomach. (P12: a daughter, aged 31–40, married, father was ill)

Almost all of the participants worked for private companies or factories, where leave requests were extremely difficult to make and rarely approved. This participant indicated that asking for leave might lead to fines or even to being laid off:

> My company also has strict rules about leave applications. Usually, we only get to go back home for the Spring Festival. I have no choice. I wanted to find work at home, but I couldn't. When this [my parent's illness] happens, even if I might get fined or lose the job, I would still come back. (P3: a son, aged 31–40, married, father was ill)

Unfinished Care and Its Impact

As reflected in the literature, political propaganda romanticises urban areas, especially the big cities, as luxury places in which to realise the 'Chinese dream' (from Chairman Xi's recent political slogan). In the meantime, anything associated with the rural is inevitably considered at least partially undesirable (Lin, 2013; Lu & Chen, 2004). A theme about travelling to the big cities as a life achievement, rooted in this idealising discourse, was spotted in participants' statements, such as this one:

> P16: After the surgery, we would like to take her to Chengdu [the provincial capital] and would be really happy if she could live longer. (P16: a son, aged 51–60, married, mother was ill)

For P16, living in rural areas symbolised hardship, sacrifice, and a lack of opportunity for relaxation and enjoyment. His perception reflected a discourse apparent in the government's modernisation project, previously discussed in Chapter 2, according to which abandoning an identity relating to rural peasantry is a meaningful and 'modern' act. Many participants expressed a sense of regret or guilt that they had not taken their parents to the big city where they worked and still wished to try and make it happen after the parent's recovery, should they recover. Instead of imagining travel to tourist locations such as scenic locations or places of cultural importance, they wanted to take their parents to the big city. This could be in part because the city is what they were familiar with; as an economically deprived group, they have few opportunities for leisure travel. If they took their parents to the city where they work, they would have more confidence in showing their parents around and also spend less money. However, their desire to show their parents the city also at least in part indicated that in the participants' estimation, urban areas offered something wonderful compared to rural areas. The following participant accounts relate to this theme of travelling.

> P1: I wish I could take him to some tourist spots or big cities by plane, but the issue is money and time. I don't have much money, and I have been quite busy with work, too. (P1: a daughter, aged 41–50, married, father was ill)

> P4: If she could walk and take the bus, I would still like to take her out to travel and see the cities. (P4: a daughter, aged 41–50, married, mother was ill)

> P6: I want to take them to many places around China. They have never enjoyed this before. (P6: a son, aged 31–40, married, father was ill)

> P24: Argh [expression of frustration]—I just wish she could recover for a bit, and then I would take her to the city so that I could take care of her. She has not been anywhere as far as I can remember. I want to take her to the city so she can know what it is like outside [the rural area where she lives]. This has always been my wish. I need to wait until she gets better. I will keep working toward that. (P24: a daughter, aged 31–40, married, mother was ill)

Being able to travel outside the rural area in which they were born was one of the most obvious differences between these participants and their parents' generation. As migrant peasant workers, participants had travelled to many big cities, even though this travel was mainly for work purposes rather than tourism. Many parents had spent almost all of their lives at home in the countryside. P3's father had also been a migrant worker when he was younger, but this participant also said, 'Even though he worked in many places, he never travelled within any of them'. Urban travel, commercial tourism, and consumerism are topics with broader connotations that go beyond the current research. However, in relation to this research, it was striking that, conscious of the limited time their parents had left to live, this became the focus of the participants' hopes for their parents. The idea of visiting the big city or taking a plane symbolically interacts with many other notions such as consumerism, and is fostered by political agendas that portray that the bigger the cities are, the merrier and fancier everything in them will be. This idea also connects with the participants' concern with attempting to appreciate the sacrifices their parents had made for the welfare of the family, as in this example:

> P21: This question really hit close to home. To be honest, I really want to take my parents to travel somewhere beautiful. I haven't travelled a lot myself. I came from a rural area, and I have to constantly worry about money. My parents wouldn't spend money on travelling even if they had any. They would spend it on us and our family. And so money is the issue for us. Health insurance could be a big issue too. (P21: a son, aged 31–40, married, father was ill)

Gender Differences in Caregiving and Care Impacts

A gendered pattern emerged in the analysis. Discourse analysis revealed that emotional burdens were more overtly expressed by daughters than sons. Sons tended to talk more about financial burdens. According to traditional filial perceptions, sons are supposed to take the main responsibility for providing financial support, daughters-in-law take charge of hands-on care, and daughters are expected to visit and to provide emotional care (Ikels, 2004). However, it was remarkably rare to see caregiving daughters-in-law in the hospital, and I was able to recruit just one daughter-in-law as a participant for this research.

When participants were asked about the gendered nature of their filial responsibilities, almost all of them initially said there should be no difference between sons and daughters in terms of taking care of parents, as illustrated in these examples:

> P3: It must be the same. Regardless of gender, as long as you truly care for your parents, I think it is all honourable. Maybe one person is more detail-oriented and emotionally sensitive than the next. In general, I didn't think one has been more caring than the other between me and my sister. We have done whatever the doctor has told us to. (P3: a son, aged 31–40, married, father was ill)

> P11: There should be no difference between sons and daughters. All children should fulfil their responsibilities. (P11: a son, aged 31–40, married, father was ill)

However, later in their interviews, some of the participants expressed there were some gender differences. The idea that 'sons are the old-age insurance' still existed. This is a popular saying, especially in rural China, and basically means sons will take care of their parents in their old age (Chou, 2011). The following participants commented on this gender issue:

> P7: In terms of this [saying], I think it's right. Generally, to raise a son is to have an old-age insurance in rural areas. I will try my best to do what I am supposed to do as a son. I am not so good, but I wouldn't be too much better or worse than others. I won't give other people the chance to judge me. (P7: a son, aged 41–50, married, father was ill)

> P19: I think sons take more [responsibility]. Daughters are already married out. (P19: a son, aged 41–50, married, father was ill)

> P20: Sons often stay with their parents. (P20: a son, aged 41–50, married, father was ill)

An interesting event occurred between a participant and her brother during one interview. When I interviewed P13, whose mother was ill, her brother (P14) entered the interview room unexpectedly. I was just asking what she thought about the difference between her and her brother's care. I did not immediately ask her brother to leave because his interview was planned to take place immediately afterwards, and because he had entered the room with the mother's doctor, with whom he engaged in discussion. I did not realise I should have asked him to leave the room until a few minutes later. Nonetheless, despite the intrusiveness of this act, an interesting scenario unfolded. P13 explained to me what she thought about the gender difference in care:

> P13: There are no differences in terms of being filial to your parents. ... There is difference in some sense [in relation to some specific tasks]. If your mother got ill, your sister would be the one to wash her because it's more convenient. It is only different because of our physical gender. (P13: a daughter, aged 31–40, married, mother was ill)

Both P13 and I thought her brother was too busy talking with the doctor to attend to what was being said. However, just after she finished her comment, he interjected in a tone and manner suggesting disagreement. He said, 'I am the son; of course I do much more than you. You are the daughter and you're already married out. I have to take care of the fees and everything; you're just providing hands-on care'. He sounded as if he was unhappy with her answer. P13 nodded without stopping. It appeared she did not want to be in conflict with her brother, and also she agreed with what he said about his financial contribution. I had to wait until he had left the room before I could continue the interview appropriately. At the end of the interview, when I asked again P13 what she thought about whether she or her sibling contributed more, she said, 'My younger brother has done more than me. He has been here all the time, and he is also around'. It seemed that her narrative was influenced by the unscheduled interruption. In the interview with the brother, held immediately after, he explained his thoughts:

> P14: My sister is married. It [the filial responsibility] has to be mine alone. She has to support her daughter. It takes a few hundred RMB to visit here. She is under a lot of financial pressure. (P14: a son, aged 31–40, married, mother was ill)

P14 thought he took most of the responsibility (mainly referring to financial responsibility) because he was the son. He took care to mention that he understood his sister's financial situation, even though he was not any better off than her and had just quit his job to come back to care for their mother; he was willing to provide the main financial support for their mother's care. This story indicated that gendered filial piety still exists.

However, the traditional gendering in filial piety has changed to a great extent. Daughters tend to take on more responsibilities for their parents. Moreover, many people are inclined to think that daughters should be no different from sons in terms of providing filial care for parents, especially when many families have just one child:

> P20: It is the same. Each one of us does their own part. It is not about how much money I spend today. If one has money, he will give more. If one doesn't have much money, he will compensate by offering other care … Nowadays, whether there are one or two children; they all have to be responsible for their parents. It is a must. Both sons and daughters need to be responsible … There is no gender difference for filial responsibilities. There is a difference in terms of children's ability and availability. Like the old saying "each of the five fingers each has its own length", some are well-off financially and some are not. Brothers and sisters need to be

> understanding of each other. (P20: a son, aged 41–50, married, father was ill)

P20 articulated a belief that children should share responsibility regardless of their gender but that they may care differently according to how close they live and how financially well-off they are. Especially under the one-child policy, whereby most families have only one child, the gender feature of filial piety has become less salient. In fact, P20 thought the difference was only attributable to financial factors, not gender.

Gendered filial practice was also still expected in relation to specific care task requirements. Most of the participants thought that hands-on care was gender-specific. As P13, a woman, explained below, sons might more appropriately provide certain types of hands-on care for the father, and daughters for the mother:

> P13: There are some things I can do for my mother that are not so convenient for him [her brother], such as bathing and toileting. (P13: a daughter, aged 31–40, married, mother was ill)

From the analysis, daughters tended to express emotional impacts more than sons did. P2 and P3, both daughters, felt prolonged distress and extreme heartbreak after their father's diagnosis. Most female participants cried or choked back tears at least once during the interview. No son showed such a reaction. P11 (a son, aged 31–40, married, father was ill) said, 'One should deal with this shift with a peaceful mind'. Or as P9 (a son, aged 31–40, divorced, father was ill) put it, 'We have to deal with the emotion when we feel it. I will try my best, anyhow'. Sons tended to express an expectation that they should be calm and in this way differed from daughters.

Additionally, some participants, such as P18 (a daughter, aged 41–50, married, mother was ill), thought that sons were not as thoughtful and detail-oriented as daughters in terms of hands-on care tasks. This sentiment was echoed by a male participant:

> P21: I think there is not much difference now from what it was before. I think daughters might be more caring than sons. Take me as an example. As a man, I have to go out and work. I can't be there to take care of my father all day, every day. Daughters are often more detail oriented and attentive in general. (P21: a son, aged 31–40, married, father was ill)

P23 was a daughter in her 20 s who had received a college education in a major city. She represented a group of migrant peasant workers who are not considered to be 'migrant peasant workers' in a traditional sense by the general public, or often, even by themselves. She offered the following conclusion:

> P23: In terms of caregiving style, I feel women are more sensitive and meticulous than men. Men are quite logical [beings] who shoulder the financial burden and handle the changes in circumstance. Of course, many only sons nowadays are quite detail oriented and sensitive, whilst some daughters are very strong-minded. I think they are the same in other aspects. Some people say there is a gender boundary, but I don't think of that as a problem. They are your parents, who just happen to be ill. (P23: a daughter, aged 21–30, single, mother was ill)

Daughters-in-law. It appeared that participants often did not take daughters-in-law into account in terms of questions around gender differences. P3 (a son, aged 31–40, married, father was ill) thought his sister's help meant more for him in terms of taking care of his father than his own wife's help. Another female participant weighed up the filial devotion between children and daughters-in-law, clearly indicating her perception that daughters-in-law are not as filial as they were in the past:

> P4: It takes up 70 –80% among children to be filial; 50% at most among daughters-in-law. (P4: a daughter, aged 41–50, married, mother was ill)

Another participant, P17 (a daughter-in-law, aged 51–60, married, mother-in-law was ill), was the only daughter-in-law participant in my research. She was quite advanced in age herself. The caregiving experience had taken a toll on her health too. She seemed able to talk about her care burden quite freely, which raises the question of whether daughters-in-law differ from children in expressing their care burden. P18, P17's sister-in-law, commented on P17's care: 'She [P17] is carrying out her duties. However, daughters-in-law can never compare to real daughters'. Daughters-in-law are not expected to devote themselves to their in-laws as they were in traditional Chinese society. To some extent this has resulted from the absolute feminism encouraged during the Mao's era. Married women were expected to stay at home and care for their parents-in-law in traditional Chinese society (Leung, 2003). In the Mao period, women were instead encouraged to work outside the home to an equal extent as men (Leung, 2003). According to the Parental Heritage Act of 1985, daughters and sons could share the inheritance from their parents equally, as opposed to the traditional norm of daughters inheriting very little or nothing (Leung, 2003). The standard for distribution of inheritance was now based on how much a child cared for the parents and no longer on gender as it had in the past, when sons inherited substantially more than daughters. With the advent of the one-child policy, daughters in a sense became sons, since there is only one child (Ikels, 2004). Thus in current Chinese society daughters-in-law are no longer expected to be the primary hands-on caregivers. This is demonstrated in P6's narrative:

> P6: My wife asked me to take good care of my father. If I need money, she'll transfer it. I didn't bring much money home, so she said she would transfer [money] if needed. (P6: a son, aged 31–40, married, father was ill)

His wife was supportive because she did not have a problem with him contributing to his parent's care. She did not express an expectation that she should be a traditional filial daughter-in-law who would take care of all the hands-on care tasks. Many other male participants also said their wives were supportive—mostly in emotional and spiritual form. None of the wives/daughters-in-law came to the hospital to care for their in-laws, apart from P17, who was of an older generation. Historical changes in gender role expectations have affected filial caregiving practices and the burdens shouldered by caregivers.

Care Responsibilities or Burdens?

According to Corlett (2016), responsibility refers to something one needs to fulfil legally or morally. Whereas a burden is a form of responsibility that is experienced as repressive and worrisome, responsibility is not necessarily a burden. Care responsibilities and burdens are often conflated terms in research on family caregivers (Dowdell, 1995; Montgomery et al., 1985; Rice et al., 1993). It is important to define and differentiate these two notions in this research since both are strongly associated with the discourse of filial piety (Zeng et al., 2014).

According to Zeng et al. (2014), Chinese family caregivers have a strong sense of responsibility for ill older parents due to the discursive influence of filial piety. However, this does not mean Chinese caregivers do not also feel a burden of care. At the beginning of their interview, every one of my participants answered that they did not think taking care of their ill parents was a burden because it was their 'natural' responsibility to provide this care. The following is an example of such a response:

> P16: When she was admitted in preparation for the surgery, my youngest sister and I were always here to take care of her. Before and after the surgery, we were both here, after then we started taking turns. In the past few days, my sister hasn't been feeling comfortable with the smells in the hospital because of her weak stomach, so she has gone back home. So I asked my wife to come. There always have to be people here. (P16: a son, aged 51–60, married, mother was ill)

P16 talked about the difficulty his sister experienced in taking care of his mother. However, he did not talk about his own difficulties. Talking about one's own difficulties in taking care of one's parents might send a message that one objects to doing so, which could be seen to be unfilial. Although early in their interviews, participants often emphasised caring for parents as a responsibility, as the end of the interview approached many began to identify the burdens they felt. Only five of the participants did not explicitly express at some point in the interview that they felt they were carrying a burden.

Speaking about a care burden could have complicated connotations. On the one hand, talking too much about experiencing caring as a burden comes across as unfilial. Hence, talking too much about physical and emotional labour might appear as if the participants were complaining about caring for their parents. Participants likely feared appearing unfilial to me. A hidden discourse was identified here; organised filial consciousness prevents people from talking too much about exhaustion and other negative impacts they felt from taking care of their parents. Such prohibitions on expressing consciousness of being tired or experiencing other negative impacts can be expected to have increased participants' emotional burden (Canda, 2013; Ott, 2003).

On the other hand, participants speaking about the sorrow they felt and reflecting on other care burdens could indicate a high level of filiality; the participants would want other people to realise what they were experiencing as it does also signify being a filial child. This recognition might also be important to participants' filial self-esteem. For example, P17 said,

> P17: Everybody in my village knows how much burden I carry, but I still paid for my mother's surgery even though I had to borrow a lot of money from people. They all know how filial I am [he smiled with a sense of pride] ... There was another guy from the village in the exact same situation last year, and he did not fulfil his [filial responsibilities]. (P16: a son, aged 51–60, married, mother was ill)

In talking about how much burden he endured, P16 was showing me and other people in his community how filial he was. This filled him with a sense of achievement and of having a 'good' reputation. Another participant also explicitly expressed the emotional burden she had carried:

> Me: Can you describe some of the ways your father's illness affects your personal life?
>
> P2: I often cry from sorrow and can barely eat. I have lost over 5 kilos in a few months. I often wake up at 1 or 2 o'clock in the morning, [and] I feel very sad thinking about my father's illness.
>
> Me: What do you find the hardest about providing care for your father?
>
> P2 [choking back tears]: The heartbreak. It feels like a hole in my heart. (P2: a daughter, aged 31–40, married, father was ill)

P2 deeply felt the anguish and pain. She cried a lot during the interview, especially when she was asked about how she felt about her father. When I asked whether she was experiencing anything positive in her current situation, she said, 'Nothing. I only feel grateful that we have fulfilled our obligations as children'. 'Nothing' here expressed quite clearly her grief and sorrow; her subsequent reference to her piety clearly delineates a relationship between filial piety and emotional stress. She felt a sense of satisfaction because she was fulfilling her obligations as a daughter. Emotional stress is a huge burden for participants. However, being steeped in sorrow and being depressed can also demonstrate (or provide evidence) that the participant is being filial. The grief emerges as a natural emotion in the participant but is also somehow required by organised filial consciousness. In a way, participants feel 'good' and relieved by feeling sorrowful because it shows they are being filial.

At times, the discourse of filial piety conflates care responsibilities and burdens. However, in identifying the subtle differences and interplay between these experiences in participants' narratives, a strong connection can be detected between the discourse of filial piety and the impacts of caregiving. Earlier, I mentioned that negative impacts on participants of their involvement in care are often associated with filial piety. In the next section, the positive role that filial piety also plays in alleviating care burdens is identified and explained.

Filial Piety as a Resource for Dealing with the Various Care Impacts and Burdens

Initially in the research proposal for this study, another form of burden was identified for exploration: the spiritual burden. However, in interviews no participant understood what spiritual meant, despite my efforts to explain. No participants or their parents appeared to belong to any organised religion. P1 explained how she tried to appeal to a higher power to help her father:

> P1: When I finally get to sleep it is past midnight. It takes about four hours for me to fall asleep, and then usually I can only sleep for three to five hours. When I go to work, I feel like I don't have as much energy as I used to. I pray to the divine that his illness will be cured, but I know it's impossible because he has a terminal illness. (P1: a daughter, aged 41–50, married, father was ill)

Religious beliefs have been suppressed to some extent in China, especially during the Cultural Revolution (Haughey, 1972; Thompson, 1984). Praying even knowing it was not possible for her prayers to be answered was a sign of P1's desperation. This was a last resort since she could not think of anything else she could do for her father to prolong his life. When I asked her later in the interview about her spiritual beliefs in relation to filial piety or her father's illness, she did not know what spirituality meant. I had to explain what religion and spirituality were, since religion has been stigmatised in China for a long period of time. I explained that religion does not necessarily mean Buddhism or Taoism or Islam but can also include beliefs around serving and respecting our parents. The participant nodded but kept silent. It seemed this question was quite difficult for her to construct an answer to.

I then asked her whether there were any spiritual benefits to her fulfilling her filial obligations. She said, 'It will enable me to be stronger when I face the obstacles life will bring me in the future. It also gives me a sense of accomplishment in terms of being a responsible child'. Giving care made her feel she was not only a responsible child but also a good person. She appeared to indicate that in fulfilling her responsibility she was spiritually reassured that she would receive similar care if in the future she encountered similar difficulties to her parent.

Instead of merely being a burden, filial piety appeared to enable participants to positively deal with other burdens of care; it functioned as a resource that might be spiritual, cultural, or philosophical. Filial piety not only helped participants to understand how they ought to resolve burdens of care but also generated a sense of pride. According to Lin (2013), this sense of occupying a cultural habitus enables migrant peasant workers to deal with their marginalised social status in the big city. Within their narratives about emotional, physical, financial, and even work-related burdens, participants always eventually related what they were saying back to filial piety. This idea resonates with scholarly contentions, such as that of Knight and Sayegh (2010), that filial piety works as a coping mechanism in Confucian cultures.

Filial Piety as a Hindrance for Dealing with the Various Care Impacts and Burdens

Filial Piety as Emotional Hindrance

When someone as close as one's parent is dying, there may be an almost universal tendency to experience fear of the loss of a sense of family wholeness (Abeles et al., 2004). Filial piety may magnify such feelings, as shown in this statement from a son whose mother was terminally ill:

> Parents are like the sky [or universe]; if the sky [the universe] falls, the family will be destroyed. (P20: a son, aged 41–50, married, mother was ill)

Another feeling was that of regret, which also appeared to be amplified by the discourse of filial piety; many participants expressed their guilt for not having done enough for their parents before the diagnosis, as did this daughter:

> I just regret I often did not do well enough in terms of fulfilling my filial responsibilities [e.g., support her mother financially and emotionally]. I don't know what I am going to do if she leaves me too soon. (P4: a daughter, aged 41–50, married, mother was ill)

Such regret or guilt was intensified by the fact that migrant workers had experienced life outside the rural area, in the metropolitan cities, but that their parents had not been able to gain such knowledge of the 'modern' world. Filial piety discursively reinforced the emergence of fear and guilt. Alleviating these feelings might attenuate the emotional distress participants experienced.

Discourse of Secrecy

The participant interviews suggested that in their understanding, and in the context of Chinese beliefs about the harm done in telling a patient about their diagnosis of cancer, filial piety was discursively translated into a series of expectations around keeping secrets. Secrets that were required to be kept included the parent's illness and the care burdens experienced by the adult child(ren).

Not Telling the Parents about the Cancer. From my participants' statements, such as the one below, it was apparent that not telling one's parent about the cancer was a common practice:

> I haven't told my father about the cancer. I fear it would add an emotional burden for him. This is the critical time when a patient needs to be mentally strong. … I persuade him to keep calm and relaxed. (P3: a son, aged 31–40, married, father was ill)

Not telling might result in additional emotional labour for the participants, as illustrated in this statement:

> We pretended nothing had happened or changed. However, when he was not around, we were so agonised that it can't be explained in words. (P1: a daughter, aged 41–50, remarried, father was ill)

To understand how this cultural practice can have come into being when Confucianism promotes parrhesia, it is necessary to consider the socially constructed nature of 'truth' and that what is considered honourable truth-telling in one culture may be considered dishonourable in another. In the Chinese context, the peace of mind of elders is considered a critical social good. The practice of not telling parents about their cancer is related to the first (complexity) and third (parrhesia) elements in the conceptual framework developed for this study. While participants adhered to the expectation that they should keep their parents' illness secret, this practice had repercussions, which are explained below.

Isolation from Friends and Colleagues. In the Confucian discourse of filial piety, a parent's death is considered an overly sensitive topic, and talking about it, even with close friends, is not encouraged. Moreover, discussing care burdens with one's friends or co-workers might be perceived as a covert request to be visited or to receive financial contributions or gifts for oneself or the ill parent.

> Interviewer: Why haven't you told others [that your parent is ill]?
>
> Participant: They have their affairs to attend to. It would add unnecessary burden for them if I told them.
>
> Interviewer: What burden?
>
> Participant: Burdens of time and money, as they might need to come to visit bearing money as a gift. (P8: a son, aged 31–40, married, father was ill)

Not telling friends or colleagues about one's emotional burden might, however, interfere with one's own processing of various forms of stress and distress. As another participant explained, if she was able to talk to her friends about her feelings about her mother's illness, she would not feel so anguished.

> All people have sad moments. If you talk it out [with friends], you will feel happier. (P2: a daughter, aged 31–40, married, father was ill)

Not Asking for Help. Discourses of filial piety dictated that the participants should accept and undertake caregiving as solely their own responsibility. As the participants below suggested, in addition to not asking for help from friends, they also thought they should not ask for help from the government.

> You can always squeeze in time even if you are super busy. ... You should not ask for help from others. Why? Because it is our filial responsibility! (P9: a son, aged 31–40, divorced, father was ill)
>
> It is our own responsibility to take care of our parents. I don't think it is the government's job to take care of them for us. (P20: a son, aged 41–50, married, mother was ill)

Conclusion

The mediating role of filial piety in participants' care experiences was multiplex and included positive and negative effects. The participants' socio-economic status as migrant workers was also strongly associated with the care burdens that they experienced and the way in which filial piety affected them. Being migrant workers could impose extra care impacts (emotional and physical impacts, financial impacts, work-related impacts, unfinished care and its impacts), which could be experienced as care burdens. Their status as migrant workers, which was the main contextual factor explored in this research, influenced participants' lived experiences through these extra care impacts. Filial piety, as the mediator for lived experiences of care, could both buffer and exacerbate care burdens. In their fulfilment of perceived filial responsibilities, filial piety helped caregivers to deal with care burdens through gaining spiritual strength. Lin (2013) claimed that this spiritual strength could produce a form of resilience, which enables migrant peasant workers to cope with their marginalised social status in the metropolitan cities, through occupying a cultural habitus and maintaining cultural capital based on filial piety. As St. André (2018) contended, filial piety emerges as a coping mechanism across all Confucian cultures when care burdens are experienced.

At the same time, filial piety could provoke stressful care experiences. This happened due to experiences of difficult emotions such as fear and guilt, emotions that were reinforced by beliefs stemming from a culture of filial piety. While fulfilling filial piety-related responsibilities provided access to resources, filial piety could also impose obstacles on migrant workers, as indicated by study participants. According to the Confucian ideology of filial piety, parents represent heaven and earth, sacrifice for one's family, and a backbone for the children (Luo, 2013); as a son earlier quoted said, 'Parents are like the sky [or universe]; if the sky [the universe] falls, the family will be destroyed'. Other participants' comments revealed a form of regret or guilt that many migrant workers might feel towards their parents for the lack of care and support they had provided before the diagnosis, especially due to their lack of proximity. Guilt is also related to the different life experiences of the participants' and the parents' generations. These life experiences had been shaped by changing socio-economic conditions and perceptions that had been encouraged to facilitate those changes. For example, as a consequence of urbanisation, participants, being migrant workers, had visited and lived in metropolitan cities. These urban experiences have been ideologically constructed as something modern, as opposed to backward and non-progressive, and therefore as something good towards which to strive (Rofel, 2007). Participants' parents were left behind at the rural home, for reasons such as old age, having to take care of grandchildren, and so on. This led to participants feeling guilty and regretful (Lin, 2013). Filial piety reinforced feelings of fear in relation to losing one's parents and regret or guilt for not providing enough care before diagnosis; thus the ideology of filial piety was implicated in increased emotional stress for migrant workers. The coexistence and interrelatedness of both the supportive and stressful effects of filial piety that were identified clearly relate to the first element of the conceptual framework, complexity, whereby the universe and the self are seen as a complex, discursive, dialectical whole.

Moreover, through the discursive construction of secrecy in the discourse of filial piety, most migrant workers carried their exceptional care burdens without access to effective support from friends, professional services, or local and national government agencies. Filial piety also translated into a discourse of secrecy through a series of discursive practices: not telling the parents about cancer, isolation from friends and colleagues, and not asking for help. Death is considered a taboo topic from the Confucian perspective. Death should not be discussed by children in front of their parents, nor should one speak of the likely death of one's parent to other people (Ikels, 2004). The discourse of filial piety also dictates that adult children not talk about their care burdens as this may risk diminishing the perception that they are filially pious (Zeng, 2012). This belief prevented participants from asking for or expecting help from others including friends, relatives, wider society, and the government. Only later in the interview, as participants became more comfortable in discussing their burdens of care, did some critique of inefficient government policies for support begin to emerge. Engaging in such critique was likely to be experienced as risky by the participants, in the first place because it might appear to diminish their filial piety, but also because many Chinese, perhaps especially rural or less educated Chinese, are fearful of the consequences of criticising the government. Researchers are not easily trusted with such confidences. Furthermore, Chinese people often find it awkward to talk about death with someone who may lose a loved one, and this discomfort applies not only to friends but also to professionals. Yet some participants overtly stated that they thought not being able to talk about a parent's impending death with friends or colleagues hindered their ability to process their emotional distress.

Additionally, only one participant told her mother the truth about her disease: that she had cancer and was terminally ill. Not informing patients that they have cancer is a common practice engaged by both medical staff and family members in China (Shi et al., 2019). Apart from the one participant, all other participants thought it important not to say anything, because to do so would most definitely decrease the remaining life expectancy of the patient by placing them under the unnecessary stress of knowing they had an incurable illness. However, while by keeping this secret participants avoided having to deal with the possible emotional breakdown of their dying parent, they also lost their chance to say goodbye and achieve emotional closure with their parent. Furthermore, although the significance of this is still not well recognised by family members and health practitioners, the ill person is left powerless in decision-making processes relating to their own health and death.

A comprehensive analysis of participants' discourses about care burdens is important, because the perception of care burdens in relation to filial piety discourse raises questions: What, if anything, has changed in terms of filial care practices? How are care practices facilitated through filial discourse despite the care burdens? In the next two chapters I explore the mechanisms that participants adopted to make sense of their subjective filial perceptions and responsibilities.

References

Abeles, N., Victor, T. L., & Delano-Wood, L. (2004). The impact of an older adult's death on the family. *Professional Psychology: Research and Practice, 35*(3), 234–239. https://doi.org/10.1037/0735-7028.35.3.234

Canda, E. R. (2013). Filial piety and care for elders: A contested Confucian virtue reexamined. *Journal of Ethnic and Cultural Diversity in Social Work, 22*(3–4), 213–234. https://doi.org/10.1080/15313204.2013.843134

Chou, R. J. A. (2011). Filial piety by contract? The emergence, implementation, and implications of the "Family Support Agreement" in China. *The Gerontologist, 51*(1), 3–16. https://doi.org/10.1093/geront/gnq059

Corlett, J. A. (2016). Responsibility. *The Journal of Ethics, 20*(1), 1–33. https://doi.org/10.1007/s10892-016-9221-1

Dowdell, E. B. (1995). Caregiver burden: Grandmothers raising their high risk grandchildren. *Journal of Psychosocial Nursing and Mental Health Services, 33*(3), 27–30. https://doi.org/10.3928/0279-3695-19950301-05

Dreyfus, H. L., & Rabinow, P. (1982). *Michel Foucault: Beyond structuralism and hermeneutics*. University of Chicago Press.

Foucault, M. (1967). *Madness and civilization: A history of insanity in the age of reason*. Tavistock.

Haughey, J. C. (1972). *Religion in Communist China* (Vol. 126). America Press.

Ikels, C. (2004). *Filial piety: Practice and discourse in contemporary East Asia*. Stanford University Press.

Knight, B. G., & Sayegh, P. (2010). Cultural values and caregiving: The updated sociocultural stress and coping model. *Journals of Gerontology Series b: Psychological Sciences and Social Sciences, 65B*(1), 5–13. https://doi.org/10.1093/geronb/gbp096

Leung, A. S. (2003). Feminism in transition: Chinese culture, ideology and the development of the women's movement in China. *Asia Pacific Journal of Management, 20*(3), 359–374. https://doi.org/10.1023/A:1024049516797

Lin, X. (2013). *Gender, modernity and male migrant workers in China: Becoming a 'modern' man*. Routledge.

Lu, M., & Chen, Z. (2004). Urbanization, urban-biased policies, and urban-rural inequality in China, 1987–2001. *Chinese Economy, 39*(3), 42–63. https://doi.org/10.2753/CES1097-1475390304

Luo, C. (2013). *Filial piety and its "Tianjingdiyi" 天经地义论孝道*. Guang Ming Ri Bao 光明日报出版社.

Montgomery, R. J., Gonyea, J. G., & Hooyman, N. R. (1985). Caregiving and the experience of subjective and objective burden. *Family Relations, 34*(1), 19–26. https://doi.org/10.2307/583753

Ott, C. H. (2003). The impact of complicated grief on mental and physical health at various points in the bereavement process. *Death Studies, 27*(3), 249–272. https://doi.org/10.1080/07481180390137044

Rice, D. P., Fox, P. J., Max, W., Webber, P. A., Hauck, W. W., Lindeman, D. A., Hauck, W. W., & Segura, E. (1993). The economic burden of Alzheimer's disease care. *Health Affairs, 12*(2), 164–176. https://doi.org/10.1377/hlthaff.12.2.164

Rofel, L. (2007). *Desiring China: Experiments in neoliberalism, sexuality, and public culture*. Duke University Press.

Shi, W., Yang, L., Liu, L., & Tan, W. (2019). 恶性肿瘤患者告知影响因素与告知模式的研究进展 [Research progress on influencing factors and patterns of informing patients with malignant tumors]. *Cancer Development, 3*, 271–276.

St. André, J. (2018). Consequences of the conflation of *xiao* and filial piety in English. *Translation and Interpreting Studies, 13*(2), 293–316. https://doi.org/10.1075/tis.00017.sta

Steigmeier, C. (1998). *Men in a cultural vise: Foucauldian genealogical analysis of the social construction of men as resistant* (Doctoral dissertation). University of Canterbury, Christchurch.

Thompson, L. G. (1984). Observations on religion in communist China: Introductory comments. *Journal of Chinese Religions, 12*(1), 33–36. https://doi.org/10.1179/073776984805308267

Zeng, L., Zhu, X. P., & Meng, X. M. (2014). Responsibility and burden from the perspective of seniors' family caregivers: A qualitative study in Shanghai, China. *International Journal of Clinical and Experimental Medicine, 7*(7), 1818–1828. http://www.ijcem.com/

Zeng, Z. (2012). Tianjingdiyi: Three phrases of philosophical argument of the validity of Confucius filial piety 天經地義:儒家「孝」道存在正當性的三次哲學論證. *Philosophy and Culture 哲學與文化, 39*, 149–169. http://lawdata.com.tw/tw/journal.aspx?no=388&pno=46184

CHAPTER 7

Parental Sacrifice Discourse

Introduction

In the previous chapter, structural changes such as urbanisation posed many challenges for adult children in terms of providing filial care for their ill parents. Participants were most concerned, however, with ensuring that their parents could enjoy as much comfort as possible before their death, and they continued to believe it was *tianjingdiyi* (natural) to take care of their parents and to be filial to them. They came back to their hometown to provide care, despite the hardships they encountered in doing so, including, for example, difficulties in taking time off work. All of the participants insisted that filial piety remained crucial for Chinese people.

As the analysis of participants' accounts unfolded, a discourse emerged that revolved around a theme of parental sacrifice. Participants thought that they were enjoying relative material abundance after the 1978 economic reform, unlike their parents before them. Participants explained their belief that their parents had made many sacrifices to raise them, and therefore they felt that in return they were morally obliged or expected to repay or make up for these sacrifices by meeting the physical, emotional, and financial needs of their parents. The discourse of parental sacrifice and the resulting adherence to ideas about filial piety served to strengthen various family and community relationship patterns. For example, fulfilling filial piety granted participants a good reputation

L. He, *Care Work, Migrant Peasant Families and Discourse of Filial Piety in China*, https://doi.org/10.1007/978-981-16-1880-2_7

within the community and also enabled them to educate the next generation (their children) about filial responsibilities. Participants' parents help raise grandchildren as a reciprocal action in exchange for filial practices.

Participants expressed several forms of emotion towards their parents and their parent's illness in the interview: fear, guilt, regret, love, and gratitude. All these emotions and the two factors mentioned above revealed the mechanism that makes sense of filial responsibilities in a changing context. Participants used this mechanism or discursive resource of parental sacrifice discourse to combat negative impacts of social changes on traditional filial practices.

Structural Changes and Power Shift

As mentioned in Chapters 1, 2, and 3, many researchers have agreed that there is a general trend towards neoliberal structural changes in, for example, family size, urbanisation, modern education, prevalence of consumerism, and mass communication (Eisenstadt, 1999). Eisenstadt (1999) claimed that even though these patterns do not constitute a transition to a simple homogenous modernity in different societies, it is essential not to ignore these neoliberal trends. Impacts of these general structural changes were reflected in my participants' statements.

Firstly, traditional large patriarchal families have been replaced by small and independent conjugal families (Ikels, 2004). According to scholars such as Fong (2006), the shrinking size of families has also been propelled largely by a one-child policy in the Chinese context. Although there is some debate about the role of the one-child policy, according to Tian (1997), there is no doubt that family size did shrink significantly after economic reform at a national level. As a result, children have to take on more caregiving responsibilities compared to previous generations (Fong, 2006). In effect, one couple becomes responsible for the care of four elders, whereas in the past several sibling couples took care of two elders (Fong, 2006).

P6 (a son, aged 31–40, married, father was ill) explained why he thought the next generation was not going to be as filial as his generation had been because the next one was the only-child generation. He pointed out the limitations of having one child who works in a city far away from his/her parents, in terms of being able to return and provide them with care. His only expectation for his daughter was to make a phone call home every now and then, rather than expecting her to come home and visit. According to Xu (2012), there has been a decrease in the frequency of children going home and visiting their rural parents. Of course, there may be other less obvious reasons for this shift in expectations. However, participants' comments indicated that the only-child generation has to bear more responsibilities than the older generation. Another participant said,

> P16: Yes, it is a bit different. It is good that our society is open since economic reform. [But] some families have elders over 70, 80 years old. All the children are away working. It is sad to see only the elders stay on at home in rural areas. This generation most often has only one child [per family]. If we get sick in the future, what can the only child do? (P16: a son, aged 51–60, married, mother was ill)

P16 indicated he felt 'sad' that people had to go out and leave their parents behind in their rural homes. However, people of his generation at least had sisters and brothers to share responsibilities. He showed his concern about the future one-child generation in terms of providing care for elderly parents as the children would have no one with whom to share caregiving tasks. P20 shared a similar concern.

> P20: I thought it was not good for my daughter to be alone. Everyone has different opinions. I fear if what happened to my eldest brother happens to me, how would my family be able to go on? (P20: a son, aged 41–50, father was ill)

The son of P20's elder brother had died in an accident. P20's sorrowful story about his nephew's death illustrated the extreme end of potential consequences of the one-child policy on family caregiving. His elder brother had no other child to provide the necessary support for him and his wife, especially as they grow older. They did not have a pension or significant savings, according to P20. In rural China, the dominant discourse of considering children (especially sons) as 'old-age security' still widely exists, especially when there is no comprehensive welfare system in place (Chou, 2011). Such events, when an only child dies from an accident or disease, raise questions and criticism about both the one-child policy and the lack of a comprehensive welfare system in China. P20 criticised the one-child policy for interfering with people's ability to secure support for their old age. Children are raised as a source of old-age care and insurance. If an only child becomes unable to provide for any reason, his or her parents will not only be devastated, they will also lose that safety net when they grow old.

Rapid urbanisation, especially after economic reform, has provided resources, benefits, and wages through the market or state benefit programmes to replace family-controlled resources. The land, which was the main resource that elders were able to trade with their children, is no longer the sole means of making a living and holds much less value than previously (Ikels, 2004). Moreover, younger generations are exposed to a wide range of ideas. They no longer need to uncritically accept ideas from their parents, including ideas regarding how to manage intergenerational relationships (Ikels, 2004). For example, they no longer strictly followed their parents' opinions about marital arrangements (Ikels, 2004).

Industrialisation and economic growth require increasing numbers of cheap workers. This has attracted rural peasants to work in urban industries (McDaniel & Zimmer, 2013). This leads to a geographical separation between migrant children and rural parents, which has made the fulfilment of filial hands-on caregiving expectations almost impossible (McDaniel & Zimmer, 2013).

Most of the participants described that they 'had to work outside [in the big cities]' even though they felt guilty leaving their parents behind in rural areas. As noted in Chapter 6 on the burden of care, almost all of the participants had to travel a long way to come back home to visit their parents. Moreover, without effective labour regulation from the government, employers exploit employees through long working hours and little job flexibility (Ikels, 2004). This lack of job flexibility, including a lack of opportunity to take leave, made it harder for participants to meet filial obligations while also working in the private labour market.

The increasing number of female workers in the market labour force has also contributed to changes in filial practices. The previous norm, according to which the eldest son's wife should live with and care for her elderly parents-in-law, appears to be weakening (Chen, 2009). According to Chen (2009), many women do not take on major care responsibilities for their parents-in-law as they did before. In ancient China, daughters-in-law stayed at home under the authority and supervision of parents-in-law, while men went out and conducted economic activities (Zhang, 2009). Since the founding of the People's Republic of China, women have been politically promoted to work (McDaniel & Zimmer, 2013). In the 1960s, 70% of urban women were working, which constituted the highest female labour participation in the world at that time. After economic reform a great need arose for a female workforce from rural areas to support the mass production industries (Zhang, 2009). The percentage of women workers have accounted for nearly 48% of workforce in China in the year 2018 (Chen, 2019). Through their employment, these rural daughters have now acquired new social roles, gained some economic independence, and increased their economic value to their parents (Zhang, 2009). The caregiving pattern has been significantly altered by this change (Cohen & Deliens, 2012). On the other hand, owing to the one-child policy, parents more evenly invest in their sons' and daughters' futures (Zhang, 2009). Daughters-in-law no longer have to stay at home and provide full-time care to their parents-in-law. They tend to be more involved in caregiving for their own parents than their parents-in-law, which counters the previous cultural norm that held that daughters only belong to their parents-in-law's family (Hooyman & Kiyak, 2008).

This social change identified in the literature was reflected in my observations during my fieldwork. I hardly ever saw a daughter-in-law (or son-in-law) taking care of the patients in the hospital. As previously noted, there was only one daughter-in-law among my participants. This participant was in her late 50s and she had retired and returned to live in her husband's family's village with her husband before her mother-in-law was diagnosed. She did have time available and it was reasonably convenient for her to actively participate in some of the hands-on care, compared to the other daughters-in-law of the patients in this research.

Participants' wives were no longer considered to be the main source of caregiving for the participants' parents. If their wives were willing and able to spend money on their parents and also to support them to return home and provide care, my participants would consider them to be supportive. Apart from these practical employment-related and geographical reasons for the absence of daughters-in-law as caregivers, Koshy (2013) argued that children are intrinsically more concerned about their own parents, partially owing to 'debt-bound value' whereby children feel morally obliged to repay a debt they owe their parents for having given them life and for raising them (Koshy, 2013). This obligation weighs especially heavily now that there are no siblings with whom to share this duty. It was evident in the field that many daughters came back to take care of their ill parents, including daughters who were not recruited for the research. Most participants, such as P11 below, thought that there should be no gender difference in terms of fulfilling filial responsibilities.

> P11: There should be no difference between sons and daughters. All children should fulfil their responsibilities. (P11: a son, aged 31–40 years, married, father was ill)

Participants' interview statements and my field observations indicated that daughters were treated as a main provider of care for parents. It did also appear that some participants still considered that sons should contribute much more financially than daughters.

Participants' stories also reflected another structural social change and associated shift in power balance.

> P21: In my parents' generation, most of them didn't have much education. They would do what their parents told them. In my generation and the next generation, public education prevails. The children know more than their parents. This has cultivated an unhealthy pride in the children. Many children don't respect their parents at all when it comes to technology and knowledge. Before, there was less money but more morality; now, there is more money but less morality. (P21: a son, aged 31–40, married, father was ill)

P21 suggested that today's younger generation tends to rebel against the older generation because the older generation has lost control over educational knowledge. The younger generation might more easily acquire knowledge than the older generation. Cohen and Deliens (2012) suggested that the increasingly wide availability of public education and public media (newspapers, television, internet, and so on) has undermined older persons' privileged position as possessors and disseminators of knowledge. As Eisenstadt (1999) stated, public education and mass media are another factor in the transformation of Chinese family values.

Many of my participants played the role of care coordinator because they knew how to manage the complicated processes involved in enrolling patients, consulting with doctors and nurses, making payments, obtaining medication, and finding places to sleep in the hospital.

Moreover, the discourse of not telling parents about the disease further indicated a widely supported belief that the younger generation held more advanced knowledge and had better decision-making capacity than the older generation. The behaviours that followed on from these beliefs reinforced knowledge inequality.

Maintained Filial Practices

Despite the potential negative influences that structural changes might have on filial perceptions and practices, my participants' stories revealed that filial practices and filial perceptions were still largely maintained. In this section, two discourses are identified to further support such maintenance of perceptions and practices: the discourses of *eat and dress well* and of what is considered *tianjingdiyi* (natural). Participants directly and specifically confirmed the presence of filial piety in themselves and in the people they knew.

Discourse of Eat and Dress Well

When participants explained their thoughts about filial piety they commonly used the phrase 'eat and dress well'. Enabling parents to eat and dress well seemed of great concern to participants.

> P1: I make his favourite food and do things with him if he wants. In other words, I am just trying to provide him with comprehensive and meticulous care (*wuweibuzhi* or *zhoudao*). I try my best to make him happy. We pretend nothing [has] happened or changed....
>
> I: When you said *wuweibuzhi*, what did you mean by that?
>
> P1: I try to make him satisfied with what he eats and wears. And I often comfort him and make him happy. (P1: a daughter, aged 41–50, remarried, father was ill)

Below are exchanges with two other participants that relate to the concept of *wuweibuzhi*. P6 said,

> P6: For me, it is to take good care of the parents—eat and dress well—and to let them enjoy life. There is nothing else.

And P12 similarly stated,

> I: Is there anything you want to do for your father but have not been able to yet?
>
> P12: I want to earn more money, so he can have a better life.
>
> I: What do you mean by a better life?

P12: To eat well and dress well. (P12: a daughter, aged 31–40, married, father was ill)

To eat and dress well literally meant enabling comfort through consuming food and through clothes. It is possible that migrant peasant workers were highly influenced by consumerism in the metropolitan cities where everything is and needs to be consumed. According to Wade (2007), commodity is the only language in the neoliberal consumerist discourse. Recent intergenerational research shows adult children are more concerned with financial exchanges than emotional and spiritual support (McDaniel & Zimmer, 2013). Neoliberal ideologies have been found to compromise emotional and spiritual support for the old (Koshy, 2013). When my participants returned home, they may bring such a perception with them. In their subjective construction of filial piety, consumerist touches penetrated and were interwoven with more traditional constructs. Therefore, being filial was to enable their parents to 'eat well and dress well'. However, it is not sufficient to only consider consumerist sources for this emphasis on eating and dressing well.

The discourse of eating and dressing well is not merely a reflection of my participants' own disadvantaged financial status; it also reflects a memory of a materially deprived past. Many of the parents continued to be significantly less well-off than their urban counterparts. According to Du et al. (2005), migration reduced rural poverty to a great extent after economic reform. However, rural areas are still not affluent by comparison with their urban counterparts (Du et al., 2005). That said, I did not detect extreme or absolute poverty during the interviews or in the questionnaire results.

Discourse of Tianjingdiyi

Another theme also emerged from participants' narrative: that of *tianjingdiyi*. The participants below all mentioned this Chinese term, which could be translated as 'natural', as also mentioned in Chapter 4.

P7: It is an unalterable fact that your parents have raised you, and it is *tianjingdiyi* that you need to be filial to them. (P7: a son, 41–50 years old, two siblings)

P8: I don't know other positive sides. It is only *tianjingdiyi* to take care of your parents. That is our tradition and value. (P8: a son, 41–50 years old, one sibling alive)

I: When was he admitted to the hospital?
P6: Last Friday.
I: When do you come here to take care of him?
P6: I am here every day.
I: Do you also sleep here at night?
P6: Yes, also here.
I: Could you describe how his disease has affected you?
P6: It hasn't had much effect.
I: No effect? What about you having to return from far away?
P6: I should come back. It is *tianjingdiyi* that I come back to be filial when parents get sick. I don't think this is a negative thing for me. (P6: a son, aged 31–40, married, father was ill)

As shown above, participants often mentioned the Chinese word *tianjingdiyi*. Being filial to one's parents was seen as the most 'natural' thing for them. The direct translation of *tianjingdiyi* is the righteousness of heaven and earth. Considering heaven and earth in Chinese fundamental philosophy stands as the root for everything (Luo, 2013), and 'natural' seems to be the English word that best translates this concept. However, what does 'natural' actually mean here? Instead of 'natural', why did I not translate this concept using a word such as 'traditional', 'moral', or 'value-laden'?

In order to understand the difference between 'natural' and these alternative terms, we need to consider the metaphysics of filial piety. Zeng (2012) thought that filial piety, as an ideology, went through three phrases. First, Confucius and his followers investigated how filial piety takes shape in an ethical sense. In the second phrase, the authors of *Xiao Jing* (孝经, *The Classics of Filial Piety*) deliberated the relationship between humans and the universe (Zeng, 2012). They claimed that filial piety was a revelation and embodiment of the universal truth (Zeng, 2012). And third, in the neo-Confucianist stage, Zhu Xi argued in favour of the justifiability and validity of filial piety at a metaphysical level (Zeng, 2012). According to Kantian scholars, a priori knowledge refers to knowledge that does not concern experience, such as truth and veridical judgements (Xu et al., 2020). However, for Zhu Xi and other neo-Confucianists, a priori knowledge and principles contained moral and ethical properties (Zeng, 2012). They rejected that morality and human ethics are produced socially, instead of holding that they are the embodiment of inner features of what was a priori (Zeng, 2012). Therefore, filial piety was not subjectively constructed in the society but rather had an objective existence that represented the truth of the universe, *tianli* (天理, Zeng, 2012). Even an animal possesses a shred of filial piety because everything is in line with the basic logic of *tianli*. According to *Zuo Zhuan* (左传, Zuo's biography), *tianjingdiyi* referred to something true that does not change or need to be challenged (Yucheng, 1992).

Thus, as P7 said, it is undoubtedly unalterable that one's parents raise one. From a discourse perspective, there are a couple of layers here. Firstly, nothing is more 'natural' than for parents to raise their children, according to neo-Confucian discourse of filial piety. Secondly, it is only fair to return the favour by being filial to parents.

Presence of Filial Perception and Filial Practice

As shown in Chapter 6, participants had experienced numerous forms of responsibilities and burdens associated with providing care to their ill parents. The extent of these responsibilities and burdens was such that they might jeopardise the realistic continuation of filial practices. The social foundation for filial piety has changed, and it was evident in participants' narratives that some practices had significantly altered as a result. For example, daughters-in-law were no longer considered to be the main provider of care for ill parents; children no longer necessarily needed to stay with parents all the time; and, at least in the hospital and health context, parents agreed that children had more knowledge than them.

Despite all of these changes, participants thought that filial piety as a morality and a collective ethic had not changed. All of the participants suggested that filial perception had not substantially changed in contemporary Chinese society, by comparison to ancient/traditional Chinese society. All participants returned to their rural homes almost immediately upon finding out about their parent's serious condition in order to provide care for the parent.

> I: Do you think there is any change now in filial perception?
>
> P1: I do not think there is too much difference between the past and the present in this.

I: What percentage of people do you think are not filial in China?

P1: Most people in China are still filial, I think. (P1: a daughter, aged 41–50, divorced, father was ill)

The above participant had been taking care of her father since his diagnosis approximately three months earlier. There was a discrepancy of sorts contained in her narrative. Earlier she said that she felt guilty about not having spent enough time with her dying father before he got sick. She expressed the thought that she was not so filial before her father was diagnosed, because she was in the city and her father lived in the rural countryside. Her work and personal life occupied most of her time. However, she did not just mention this to me as if she thought she was not filial. To admit her guilt was, in a paradoxical way, to show that she was still filial at heart. While she had experienced difficulties in providing increased care to her father, this did not mean she did not know what she 'should' do. Filial piety in traditional China represents something good, noble, and admirable (Zeng, 2012). The contextual changes that are taking place in China allow people to justify not totally following the laws of filial piety, but this does not mean that people no longer consider filial piety to be an expression of high morality.

Children were the primary caregivers in the hospital, due to a shortage of doctors and nurses in the hospital in which I undertook my fieldwork (as is commonly the case in Chinese hospitals). This applied to every participant in my study. While undertaking my fieldwork, I observed only one patient who did not have any family members with her when she received her chemotherapy. I spoke with her for half an hour. She told me that her son was working in a bigger city. She did not want him to return from the city to care for her because she wanted him to be able to focus on his career and his own life. Unlike my participants, the patient was an urban resident. Although she said this, I could see her disappointment and I noticed her insecurity as she was trying to explain this to me. It seemed as if she felt embarrassed about the fact that her son was not there to be filial to her. Her embarrassment suggested that not being cared for by family members was an uncommon phenomenon in the hospital where the field study was undertaken. When I asked participants to estimate what percentage of Chinese people might be unfilial, only one person estimated this at more than 30%. The rest of my participants considered there was less than 10%, or even 1% of people in China who were unfilial.

They thought filial practices still predominated in Chinese families. As P3 said,

> P3: Most people are still filial in China. (P3: a son, aged 41–50 years old, married, father was ill)

Taken together, these examples suggest that the discourse of filial piety continues to exist and play an important role in Chinese rural families.

Emerging Theme: Sacrifice

As mentioned in Chapter 3, in everyday life, the flow of power and responsibilities between parents and children is not balanced. The child generation tends to exercise more power than the parent generation. Parents provide much more care to their children and their children's children than children provide to their parents in old age. The discourse of filial piety to an extent appears to be an attempt to reduce this imbalance by encouraging a reciprocal relationship between children and parents and encouraging children to feel gratitude and return favours to their parents. Filial piety was built on the notion of balancing the flow of intergenerational care and interactions, which embodies socially constructed humanity.

The extent to which filial practices were maintained by participants demonstrates that people's values and moral beliefs can adapt to contextual changes. As a matter of fact, filial piety has constantly evolved throughout history. As discussed previously in Chapter 2, in the nineteenth and early twentieth centuries, the traditional culture of Confucian filial piety faced a major setback. The New Culture Movement started to denigrate Confucianism and to label feudal ethics as being cannibalistic (Ikels, 2004). After that, Chinese people witnessed the destruction of Confucianism and filial piety during the Great Leap Forward (GLF) (1958–1962) and the Cultural Revolution (CR) (1966–1976) (Yan, 1999). The discourse of highly criticising filial piety during the New Culture Movement, GLF, and CR constituted a break from earlier traditions, and is also discontinuous with the current discourse that encourages a revival of filial piety. However, the current (re)construction of filial discourse requires this discontinuity to be obscured. My analysis identified a discursively formed direct and linear linkage and connection between the present and the recent past. This connection was seen to be constructed through parental sacrifice discourse, distilled from participants' narratives.

The centrality of themes of sacrifice first appeared in narratives focusing on the participants' own experiences. This is reflected in the comment made by P6 below, also cited earlier in this chapter (on the discourse of *tianjingdiyi*).

> I: Could you describe how his disease has affected you?
>
> P6: It has not affected me much.
>
> I: No effect? What about you having to come back from far away?
>
> P6: I should come back. It is *tianjingdiyi* that I come back to be filial when parents get sick. I don't think this is a negative thing for me. (P6: a son, aged 31–40 years old, married, father was ill)

P6 said that his father's disease had no effect on him because he *should* come back to give care. In doing so he was thus just following the universal truth or the natural path. The concept of parental sacrifice next emerges when the same participant emphasised how much hardship his father had endured and how many sacrifices his father had made for him and his family during 'those years' (indicating the years of the CR). This perception of his father's sacrifice helped the participant to reciprocate by taking care of his father, despite all the challenges and obstacles he faced, such as remote location and difficulty taking leave from work. Participants' narratives of sacrifice elicited balancing narratives of parental sacrifice into the equation. Parental sacrifice discourse refers to the belief that parents have made a great many sacrifices for their children and must be repaid. The construction of parental sacrifice enables one's adaptability in response to contextual changes that threaten to constrain filial practice. This theory emerged from the data and will be explained in the following sections of this chapter.

Personal Gain

Fulfilling filial piety provided participants with personal rewards, such as an opportunity to educate the next generation to be filial through modelling being a good child and enhancement of their own reputation within their communities. Almost all of the participants believed providing care for their parents included an educational purpose for their own children. By the same logic, they believed that if people do not fulfil their responsibilities, their children will in turn neglect to care for them when they grow old. Filial piety, according to the participants, was a legacy that needs to be passed on from one generation to the next.

> P7: All of us have children too. We need to set a good example for them. (P7: a son, aged 41–50, married, father was ill)

Another participant also commented,

> P9: I have always known that I am doing this for my children too. We should educate them by setting good examples. I haven't thought about other benefits. (P9: a son, aged 31–40, divorced, father was ill)

And another said,

> P17: We all get old someday; we need to set good examples for the next generation. (P17: a daughter-in-law, aged 51–60, married, mother-in-law was ill)

Some participants, such as P14, noted that they had also learnt how to take care of their parents from their experiences of their own parents' hands-on caring. Therefore, the skills of filial care were passed on from generation to generation. The best education the participants could provide for their children was to provide good examples in their own behaviours.

Secondly, as discussed earlier in this chapter, and also as P14 below claimed, fulfilling filial piety continued to be a moral virtue, which enabled participants to accrue a good reputation.

> P14: If we don't do it well, people will talk and say you are unfilial. Most people would be afraid of such negative talk. (P14: a son, aged 41–50, married, mother was ill)

Fulfilling such an important moral duty would undoubtedly bring advantages for individuals. According to P16 below, providing care and financial assistance to his mother brought him respect from his relatives and neighbours.

> P16: I think all are important for me. Because the relatives think I am filial, they respect me for that. (P16: a son, aged 51–60, married, mother was ill)

He was smiling with obvious pride when he said this to me. Sitting near him, I could discern that he was very proud to fulfil his filial responsibilities and very content with the good reputation doing so had brought him. Especially when he talked about other people in his village who did not fulfil their filial responsibilities, his tone indicated that he felt himself to be on higher moral ground. He appeared to look badly upon those who failed to be filial children.

Reciprocity

As mentioned in the previous section, participants had personal reasons for fulfilling their filial responsibilities. Their parents also facilitated and strengthened the filial bond between generations through providing incentives (such as helping raise grandchildren). This suggested a reciprocal relationship.

The filial system, traditionally and still today, depends on parents for stability and protection. In current Chinese society, parents are an important source of support for the rearing of grandchildren and for meeting financial needs (Burnette et al., 2013). According to reports by the China Research Centre on Ageing, 35.38% of older people in rural areas contributed to raising their grandchildren in 2006 (Burnette et al., 2013). Under the traditional filial norm, children are required to put their parents' wishes and demands above other responsibilities (Canda, 2013). There were no formal obligations for grandparents in traditional Chinese society in terms of rearing grandchildren (Chen et al., 2011). However, it has become increasingly common for grandparents to help raise grandchildren both in rural and urban China (Canda, 2013). This indicates that recent social transformations have had an impact on patterns of filial practices, and that people have adapted to these changes in ways that continue to strengthen familial ties. While the form and content of familial relationships have changed, these adaptations to change echo those made to maintain strong ties between children and parents historically.

Grandparenthood is regarded as a coping strategy to maximise the whole family's well-being. For my participants, due to this support, the parents of the grandchildren, especially the mother, were enabled to go to larger cities to pursue work and hence enhance the family's economic welfare without having to worry about their child. F. Chen et al. (2011) suggested that when grandparents provide care for grandchildren, this acts as a bargaining chip which they may later exchange for receiving care in old age. For the participant quoted below, as for several other participants, his parents had helped raise his children. He worried what would happen now that his parents were no longer available to carry out this grandparenting role.

> P22: My parents have practically been raising my children for me, and I cannot ask them to help me raise my children anymore because of this [illness]. (P22: a son, aged 31–40, remarried, father was ill)

As P22 suggested, he might lose the ability to go out to work because his parents were no longer able to raise their grandchildren. In some cases, the patients were also migrant peasant workers, just like their adult children. P3 below mentioned that one of the negative impacts of his father's illness was the loss of an additional source of income for the whole family. For P3, his father's income was an important financial resource for his family. If his father could no longer work, the participant would have to earn more to support his family.

> P3: It definitely has a lot of impacts. For example, when my father was still well, he could earn money instead of spending money now. Because my father was an accountant for many years, his income was stable and handsome. (P3: a son, aged 31–40, married, father was ill)

These comments from participants indicated that parental sacrifice was not merely imagined. There is no doubt that these participants' parents made actual sacrifices to support their adult children and their grandchildren. The father of P3 did not only pursue financial gain for his own benefit but also for that of his adult children and their families. Some of the participants still partially depended on their parents financially. As migrant workers, they minimised their food expenses to save money. Their parents would send them meat from the slaughter of domestic animals, food they had purchased, or vegetables they had grown. P9 below described this kind of practice.

> P9: In the summer, after they harvested rice [and sell it], they would buy me 50 or 60 chickens [with the money they got from selling the rice]. (P9: a son, aged 31–40, divorced, father was ill)

A gendered pattern was also discerned in the comments of the following two male participants. For both these participants it was their fathers who were ill. Both saw the figure of the father as the pillar of the family. As one of them said:

> P3: A family has to have a father. My father's illness has had a huge negative impact on my mother, me and my sister. As children, we wish he could live a long and healthy life. Without one parent, the family feels incomplete. Humans have emotions, unlike grass or wood. While he is alive, everything is peaceful and complete. When he is gone, something will be missing. (P3: a son, aged 31–40, married, father was ill)

Another participant also commented:

> P11: Try to think about it. If you lost the 'family master', you have to shoulder everything by yourself.... Before, my parents [would take] care of everything. For example, only they know how to do farming work; I need to go out and earn money. What will happen to my child and mother without my father? All of these questions just came into my head; there has to be that moment when you can actually think about these questions. (P11: a son, aged 31–40, married, father was ill)

There is an old Chinese saying: 'When the man of a family falls down, the family becomes incomplete'. The participant statements above suggested that the speakers, originally from rural China, adhered to relatively traditional patriarchal notions of the father. The devoted care parents had provided, and the sacrifices they had made for their children and their children's children, stimulated the participants to return home to provide care for their parents when they became ill. The nature of intergenerational relationships was reciprocal in this way. Sacrifice came from both sides. Caring for parents was also about ensuring that the participants' children might adopt and pass on filial piety in their turn, in an attempt to secure the continuation of this cycle of reciprocity.

Respect, Fear, Regret and Guilt, Love, Gratitude, and Sacrifice

Person-to-person emotional relationships can reach profound levels (van Schaik & van Noordwijk, 1982). According to van Schaik and van Noordwijk (1982), these relationships deepen over time along three dimensions—the past, present, and future—and feelings such as fear, guilt, and love are generated through interactions within and across these three dimensions. Carstensen et al. (1999) emphasised that perceptions of time are fundamentally involved in the generation of emotions. Present emotions are generated through imagined pasts and futures. From a Foucauldian perspective, pasts are perceived and futures are imagined through present discourses (Elden, 2002). This idea is central to sacrifice theory. Sacrifices that children 'remembered' their parents as having once made resulted in their need to be grateful. In their memories, they 'knew' how dependent they once were on their parents. In their consciousness of a future dimension of time, they 'knew' that what they did now would affect their own children's filial behaviours.

Respect. As shown below, for the participants, losing one's parent was not solely about losing someone for oneself. It was also about losing a family member on whom others had become dependent. As P11 was earlier quoted to have said,

> P11: Try to think about it. If you lost the 'family master', you have to shoulder everything by yourself. (P11: a son, aged 31–40, married, father was ill)

P20 similarly explained that the wholeness of the family would be no more if his father were to die.

> P20: I wish my parents could live up to be 100 years old. Everyone wants their family to be united. If there is one gone, there will be a hole in our heart for at least five years after. (P20: a son, aged 41–50, married, father was ill)

Fear. For P20, the anticipated loss was not only the loss of a sense of family wholeness. The loss of the father would result in the loss of generational interdependency, which was scary for the participant. P20 said, 'Parents are like the sky (heaven); if the sky falls, the family will be destroyed'. P3 described how he mentally depended on his father:

P3: I depend on him mentally ... I don't know what to do without him for this family. (P3: a son, aged 41–50, married, father was ill)

The perception of extreme parental sacrifice also constructs the context in which a fear of losing the support and contributions of parents arose and was intensified. For participants such as P20 and P3, the fear was so strong that I could see this reflected in their faces during the interviews.

Regret and Guilt. The fear of losing someone they could depend on induced another feeling: regret. This feeling was widely evident among my participants. Many of them regretted that they had not done enough for their parents before their parents' diagnosis, as shown in the statements below, and were fearful about their parents' impending death: they would not have any more chances to be filial 'enough' to their parents after they died. Regret could also involve feelings of guilt.

For example, P4 (a daughter, aged 41–50, married, mother was ill) could not hold back her tears when she remembered the devotion her mother had shown towards her, which was expressed in raising the participant's children, and supporting her emotionally and materially. The fear of losing her mother and the guilt of not having been more filial to her was evident in her words. Later in the interview she said, 'I just regret I often did not do well enough [e.g., support her mother financially and emotionally] by her. I don't know what I am going to do if she leaves me too soon'.

Other participants also expressed regret.

I: Do you ever behave with your mother in ways that you later regret?

P14: There are [things I regret from] before she got ill. (P14: a son, aged 31–40, married, mother was ill)

I: Have you ever done anything to your mother/father that you later regretted?

P22: Not since his diagnosis. However, I wish I could have been there for him when his diagnosis was made, but I have to earn money. (P22: a son, aged 31–40, re-married, father was ill)

P3: I have always respected my father. I have never complained or held grudges towards him, even when I got beaten as a kid. He has done a lot [for the family]. People need to put themselves into other people's shoes too, everything he has done is for this family. But sometimes I do have regrets. I started to work in the same the department where he was working when I was young. I couldn't finish my tasks well at all, and I was naughty too. I never thought about sending money home at that time. I had no sense of responsibility at that time. I only became sensible after I got married. I felt I did let him down in front of his colleagues and superiors. I feel guilty about it. (P3: a son, aged 41–50, married, father was ill)

P3 expressed regret because he had not worked hard when he was younger. Saving face is one of the most important components of being filial. P3 felt guilty not only because he brought shame on his father but also because he failed to meet his father's expectations and appreciate his love. In the participant's mind, his father had done a lot for his family and for him, and yet he brought shame on his father. Participants like P3 expressed deep guilt because their parents made great sacrifices for them, which they felt they did not sufficiently repay.

Love. A term in Chinese that does not have an equivalent translation in English is *teng ai* (疼爱), meaning literally 'painful love'. It refers to love so strong that it brings physical pain. Love or *teng ai* was not mentioned directly in the conversations between participants and me.

I: Has your relationship with your father changed since he was diagnosed with cancer?

P3: My father doesn't speak too much, just like me. My whole family is not talkative, but we all understand how much we mean to each other. My father only does things. I don't express my feelings to him either. I feel like our family is not [a proper family] if any one of us is missing, especially this year because my father got sick a lot. I depend on him mentally and emotionally. His disease is having a major effect on my mother. She desperately hopes he can recover. My father has had a hard life. He couldn't even get enough food to eat before. You might not know this because you are still young. When we were little, we had to save everything just to get by. Now we are better off and have purchased a house in the city [Langzhong]. He has a grandson too. He can finally enjoy his life, but this happens. What a storm to arise from a clear sky!

I: So after he got ill, memories appeared in your mind.

P3: Even though we don't talk that much, we all understand. So these scenes always linger in my mind. (P3: a son, aged 41–50, married, father was ill)

P3 above was in his late 30s. Apparently, he did not tell his father that he loved him and that he depended on him. He thought his father and the rest of the family knew that already. Love was something that went without saying, for him. It appeared to be almost awkward to say words like 'love'. He presumed that other people understood his feelings towards them. Filial piety does not demand that people express things verbally but rather through actions (Feng, 1995; Gao, 1998). Nonetheless, this does not necessarily mean that filial piety requires hands-on care over non-material and emotional care. In the logic of filial piety, love towards one's parents is something natural (*tianjingdiyi*), which already exists in the universe even before one is born (see Chapter 2).

Articulating love for family members takes away the power that the narrative of love possesses, to some extent. Burying it deep down in one's heart is considered to be a mature and honourable practice, especially among men. P3 said, 'You might not know this because you are still young'. Even though he was talking about how harsh living conditions were in 1960s and 1970s, when I was not yet born, he also meant I might not be mature enough to understand that deeply buried love. The marker of one's maturity is widely considered to be the ability to truly understand, be grateful to, and love one's parents without needing to verbalise it. Following that, love comes with the practice of caring and putting parents' wishes and interests above one's own. This is deemed to be much more powerful and mature than saying 'I love you' to one's parents.

Gratitude. The importance of being grateful for parental sacrifices also emerged directly from the participants' comments, such as this one:

> P20: Firstly, besides the financial side, every child needs to be filial. Parents have raised you; you need to repay the favour when they become old [foremost by being grateful]. It is natural. His disease has put emotional pressure on me. (P20: a son, aged 41–50, married, father was ill)

Twenty-two out of 24 participants described their parents as having had a life of *xinku* (辛苦, hardship). All of them explicitly or implicitly indicated the sacrifices their parents had made for the welfare of their family and expressed their gratitude for these sacrifices that had been made despite the hardships their parents had faced. The following comments from various participants illustrate this gratitude.

P1: He always puts his children's needs first. (P1: a daughter, aged 41–50, remarried, father was ill)

P12: Their generation's life was so hard and bitter. We expected they could enjoy their lives for a few of years. Even though medical technology is pretty advanced nowadays, this is not some minor issue. Therefore, I haven't been able to accept this emotionally. Yes, the surgery costs a lot of money; it creates a big financial burden. (P12: a daughter/only child, aged 31–40, married, father was ill)

P13: Yes. She was *xinku* when she raised my child. Even when we went back home, she would be the one to cook for us [choking and sobbing]. (P13: a daughter, aged 31–40, married, mother was ill)

P16: As children, we consider my mother did not have it easy raising us, especially in 'those years' [Cultural Revolution]. She also raised our children. We feel that she has suffered a lot in her life. We need to step up and be filial to her now. (P16: a son, aged 51–60, married, mother was ill)

P19: How do I put it ... my father cannot do much work such as the heavy lifting and growing crops that he used to do. They have had many years of the hard life. You know how hard it was in those years.... As their son, I should do my part. I want them to rest for a few years. Maybe when he gets better, he can keep some chickens and ducks. I hope he can live a few years.... I adore and feel for them. Their life was really hard when they were young. (P19: a son, aged 41–50, married, father was ill)

The participants' descriptions of their parents' lives as involving extreme hardship and sacrifice indicated their gratitude. This gratitude was embodied in their end-of-life care for their parents. The actions of care emerging from gratitude closely related to the discourse of *tianjingdiyi*. Because of the hardship their parents had endured and the sacrifices they had made, the children were able to grow up. Therefore, the participants needed to be grateful for their parents' sacrifices.

P7: Because the material conditions are so good now, they don't know how the older generation lived. They have forgotten about many things. Our father's generation told us about things such as Cultural Revolution, the commune, and what they suffered then. (P7: a son, aged 41–50, married, father was ill)

P7's parents' generation had told him how hard life was during the GLF and CR, so his generation still knew of the hardships their parents had endured back then. Therefore, they needed to be filial to their parents. P7 suggested the younger generation did not know about or had forgotten the harsh times that existed in 'those years'.

P7 raised a question concerning whether the generation following his would be grateful and filial or not. From his perspective, gratitude had to be based on whether or not one's parents had endured harsh times in their lives. If parents make sacrifices, then it follows that children will repay these sacrifices. If parents do not make sacrifices, or children are unaware of their sacrifices, then children may not feel as obliged to reciprocate.

Other Forms of Parental Sacrifice

> P12: I had to pressure him until he finally agreed to be admitted to the hospital ... because he does not want us to be too financially burdened. (P12: a daughter, aged 31–40, married, father was ill)

For P12 above, cancer was a disease that could change not only the patient's life but also the lives of family members. Some of the participants' parents initially did not want to go to the hospital because they did not want to spend too much money, especially knowing that their children would struggle to pay for their hospitalisation and medical care. The sacrifices made by parents did not end with the end of the CR. The participants' parents continued to make sacrifices. For participants, their perception of their parents' sacrifice was not based on tales of past events but on actions existing in their lived experiences. Some parents were determined to provide for and devote themselves to their children. Therefore, when they found that there was something physically wrong with their body, their children had to persuade them to go to the hospital and to not worry about the costs involved. This seemed to be a pattern that was almost fixed, because almost every participant described a similar process having unfolded. Several participants explained that even if their parents wanted to go to the hospital and receive treatment, they still seemed to need to initially reject hospitalisation because they needed to maintain the image of being a good parent. The parents had a tendency to maintain the parental sacrifice discourse for their children, in a similar vein to how they had told hardship stories to their children when they were little, as a reminder. By behaving in a manner that might at first appear illogical because they went against their own wish to be taken care of medically, the parents ensured that both parties could have their needs met: parents could appear to be understanding and virtuous, sacrificing their lives for their children, while the children could appear to be filial by contributing financially and emotionally and caring solely about their parent's health. There was a mutual discourse about this ritually approved sacrifice.

Conclusion

As discussed above, after the economic reforms starting in 1978, many rural residents left for big cities to make a living. Adult children no longer lived with their parents. Moreover, because of the social and technological changes that ensued, such as access to public education and the internet, the knowledge parents held was not valued as much within the modern context. There was a discernible intergenerational power shift. Contextual changes affected cultural and social values and placed enormous challenges on the maintenance of filial values and practices. These challenges were evident in participants' narratives about their caregiving for their ill parents. However, participants' narratives also showed that filial practices still widely prevailed and filial values were still highly praised. To elucidate how participants constructed filial piety in the context of social, cultural, and economic shifts in current Chinese society, participants' narratives were analysed closely until an underlying discourse emerged.

Discerning a discourse of parental sacrifice provided a means for understanding mechanisms involved in maintaining filial piety in its present context. The discourse of parental sacrifice served as a glue to connect different discourses and sub-discourses. Its discovery was directly derived from participants' narratives. These narratives asserted that parents had been continuously making sacrifices, in the participants' subjective constructions. Therefore, they needed to provide filial care in return. Parents' past sacrifices induced memories in the children relating to the very important historical period of the CR (as well as the GLF for some older participants). This was a time, according to some of my participants, when their parents endured extreme hardship and made extraordinary sacrifices in order to raise their children. This conceptualisation of sacrifice discourse raised questions in relation to history and time. How did participants make sense of filial piety today in terms of the past?

From a Foucauldian perspective, time does not flow linearly, and pasts are imagined through present discourses. In the next chapter, I will discuss the discursive formation of the past through the lens of my participants' narratives of the present. Participants' imagination of parental sacrifice during the GLF and the CR revealed another underlying discourse—the discourse of forgetting. The discourse of forgetting entwined with not only participants' subjective construction of filial responsibilities but also political and public discursive formations and influences.

References

Burnette, D., Sun, J. J., & Sun, F. (2013). A comparative review of grandparent care of children in the U.S. and China. *Ageing International, 38*(1), 43–57. https://doi.org/10.1007/s12126-012-9174-z

Canda, E. R. (2013). Filial piety and care for elders: A contested Confucian virtue reexamined. *Journal of Ethnic and Cultural Diversity in Social Work, 22*(3–4), 213–234. https://doi.org/10.1080/15313204.2013.843134

Carstensen, L. L., Isaacowitz, D. M., & Charles, S. T. (1999). Taking time seriously: A theory of socioemotional selectivity. *American Psychologist, 54*(3), 165–181. https://doi.org/10.1037/0003-066X.54.3.165

Chen, F. N., Liu, G. Y., & Mair, C. A. (2011). Intergenerational ties in context: Grandparents caring for grandchildren in China. *Social Forces, 90*(2), 571–594. https://doi.org/10.1093/sf/sor012

Chen, S. (2009). Aging with Chinese characteristics: A public policy perspective. *Ageing International, 34*(3), 172–188. https://doi.org/10.1007/s12126-009-9043-6

Chen, Y. (2019). *Female labor participation rate and influence factors in China 中国城镇女性劳动参与率影响因素研究* (Doctoral dissertation). Guizhou University, Guiyang.

Chou, R. J. A. (2011). Filial piety by contract? The emergence, implementation, and implications of the "Family Support Agreement" in China. *The Gerontologist, 51*(1), 3–16. https://doi.org/10.1093/geront/gnq059

Cohen, J., & Deliens, L. (2012). *A public health perspective on end-of-life care*. Oxford University Press.

Du, Y., Park, A., & Wang, S. (2005). Migration and rural poverty in China. *Journal of Comparative Economics, 33*(4), 688–709. https://doi.org/10.1016/j.jce.2005.09.001

Eisenstadt, S. N. (1999). *Fundamentalism, sectarianism, and revolution: The Jacobin dimension of modernity*. Cambridge University Press.

Elden, S. (2002). *Mapping the present: Heidegger, Foucault and the project of a spatial history*. A&C Black.

Feng, Y. (1995). *History of Chinese philosophy 中国哲学史*. Zhonghua Shuju.
Fong, V. L. (2006). *Only hope: Coming of age under China's one-child policy*. Stanford University Press.
Gao, G. (1998). "Don't take my word for it": Understanding Chinese speaking practices. *International Journal of Intercultural Relations, 22*(2), 163–186. https://doi.org/10.1016/S0147-1767(98)00003-0
Hooyman, N. R., & Kiyak, H. A. (2008). Opportunities and challenges of informal caregiving. In N. R. Hooyman & H. A. Kiyak (Eds.), *Social Gerontology: A Multidisciplinary Perspective* (pp. 385–428). Allyn & Bacon.
Ikels, C. (2004). *Filial piety: Practice and discourse in contemporary East Asia*. Stanford University Press.
Koshy, S. (2013). Neoliberal family matters. *American Literary History, 25*(2), 344–380. https://doi.org/10.1093/alh/ajt006
Luo, C. (2013). *Filial piety and its "Tianjingdiyi" 天经地义论孝道*. Guang Ming Ri Bao 光明日报出版社.
McDaniel, S., & Zimmer, Z. (2013). *Global ageing in the 21st Century: Challenges, opportunities and implications*. Ashgate.
Tian, X. (1997). Sustainable development of the population, the economy and the environment. *China Social Science: English Version 中国社会科学: 英文版* (3), 29–35. http://www.cqvip.com/QK/85892X
van Schaik, C. P., & van Noordwijk, M. A. (1982). Social stress and the sex ratio of neonates and infants among non-human primates. *Netherlands Journal of Zoology, 33*(3), 249–265. https://doi.org/10.1163/002829683X00110
Wade, R. H. (2007). Globalization as the institutionalization of neoliberalism: Commodification, financialization, and the anchorless economy. In W. R. Garside (Ed.), *Institutions and market economies: The political economy of growth and development* (pp. 250–277). Palgrave Macmillan. https://doi.org/10.1057/9780230389946
Xu, J. (2012). Filial piety and intergenerational communication in China: A nationwide study. *Journal of International Communication, 18*(1), 33–48. https://doi.org/10.1080/13216597.2012.662466
Xu, J., He, L., & Chen, H. (2020). Balancing instrumental rationality with value rationality: Towards avoiding the pitfalls of the productivist ageing policy in the EU and the UK. *European Journal of Ageing, 17*(2), 251–257. https://doi.org/10.1007/s10433-019-00527-9
Yan, J. (1999). Evaluation of the argument between "4th May", "Cultural Revolution" and the traditional culture 评 "五四", "文革" 与传统文化的论争. *Chinese and Foreign Culture and Discussion 中外文化与文论, 1*(2), 2–13. http://www.gwyoo.com/qikan/zhengfawenshi/wenhua/201003/354695.html
Yucheng, S. (1992). *Chunqiu Zuo's documentary 春秋左传学史稿*. Jiangsuguji Publisher 江苏古籍出版社.

Zeng, Z. (2012). Tianjingdiyi: Three phrases of the philosophical argument of the validity of Confucius filial piety. 天經地義:儒家「孝」道存在正當性的三次哲學論證. *Philosophy and Culture 哲學與文化, 39*, 149–169. http://lawdata.com.tw/tw/journal.aspx?no=388&pno=46184

Zhang, G. (2009). A study of the Taoist attitude toward the doctrine of filial piety 道家孝道思想研究. *Yuxi Normal College Journal 玉溪师范学院学报* (2), 10–15. http://xuebao.yxnu.net/

CHAPTER 8

Intertwined Discourse of Parental Sacrifice and Forgetting

Introduction

The last chapter explored a discourse of parental sacrifice that emerged in the participants' interviews. In this chapter, another discourse is highlighted, that of forgetting, which was found to be very much intertwined with the parental sacrifice discourse. The various dimensions of forgetting discourse are covered in two main chapter sections, covering filial forgetting and (political and) public forgetting. The section on filial forgetting is focused on participants' personal and subjective views of the past, mainly the periods of the Great Leap Forward (GLF; 1958–1962) and the Cultural Revolution (CR; 1966–1976). The section on public forgetting considers public agendas including how participants feel about the 'parent-visiting law'.

Although separately presented in the chapter, filial forgetting and public forgetting discourses are interwoven rather than occurring in isolation from one another. This interweaving of the two discourses was particularly evident in the analysis of participants' interviews, where the political and public discourse on forgetting could be seen to exert a major influence over participants' individual construction of forgetting discourse. The analysis of relevant policy documents and academic literature supported the identification of a public discourse of forgetting, but, although this public discourse appeared to be in response to social

L. He, *Care Work, Migrant Peasant Families and Discourse of Filial Piety in China*, https://doi.org/10.1007/978-981-16-1880-2_8

changes, it was less obviously directly influenced by the experiences of individuals such as the caregiver participants in my research.

The Foucauldian notion of power nevertheless identifies that power exists everywhere (Foucault, 1972). For Foucault, power was not limited to institutional power. Dominated individuals and oppressed social groups have their own resilience, and power can be practised both by them and by institutions (Foucault, 2000). Traditional understandings of power suggest that power can only be exercised by A over B or that power is held by a dominant group which exerts it over the dominated, either overtly or covertly (Foucault, 2000). However, Foucault did agree that governmental power is very important within the discursive formation of any given culture (Foucault, 2000). Institutional power held by the government plays an important role in a relatively top-down nation such as China. It is therefore crucial to include and understand institutional power and its impact on participants' discursive formation. Equally importantly, it is vital to bear in mind that other forms of power also shape the formation of various discourses, such as neoliberal market forces, economic convenience, and social practices in particular health settings. This book sought to understand the discourse of filial piety through migrant peasant workers' explanations of their experiences in an end-of-life care setting in the Chinese context. Therefore the discussion of power in this thesis is mainly focused on that purpose of understanding filial piety.

Filial Forgetting

As explained in the previous chapter, almost every participant mentioned the hardships their parents had endured when their parents were much younger. Participants only remembered their parents' lives as having been filled with sacrifice and extreme difficulties, especially during the GLF and the CR. Constructing such memories required a discourse of forgetting. A discourse of forgetting allowed participants to maintain a parental sacrifice discourse by failing to recall contradictory events and behaviours. These overlooked events and behaviours included their parents' past defiance of filial piety during the GLF and CR when filial piety was denigrated as something backward and repressive, and the self-serving aspects of their parents' sacrifices for their children, which were expected to be repaid in the parents' old age. This is not to say that my participants' parents did not suffer material deprivation during the time of the GLF and CR or that they did not devote their lives to service to their families, but rather that the discourse of forgetting was a mechanism or discursive resource that served to maintain the present, single-minded discourse of filial piety.

Remembering and Forgetting Parental Sacrifice

Rofel (2007) adopted the discourse of remembering and forgetting to understand three generations of female workers in a textile factory in China, in her book *Desiring China: Experiments in Neoliberalism, Sexuality, and Public Culture*. She identified a narrative/discourse of forgetting in the stories of her youngest participants (born in the 1970s, just before economic reform in 1978) and from her own observations. This generation forgot how their parents once worked for 'noble' ideological ideals and only remembered the hardships their parents and grandparents endured during the GLF and CR (Rofel, 2007). During the GLF and CR, China was closed to outside influences and strongly focused on ideological perceptions (Rofel, 2007). Then from 1978, when the economic reforms commenced, that earlier period of time had to be substantially dismissed and forgotten to facilitate economic reform. Rofel explained her findings by drawing on the concept of forgetting discourse. Rofel made sense of her participants' construction of modernity by explaining that they remembered the GLF and CR as a period of extreme suffering and unrelenting hardship. According to Rofel, both the government and the public arena promoted this discourse about the GLF and CR to legitimise economic reforms and open up to the global world (including the market) in 1978. In my research, drawing on Rofel's concept, I also identified a discourse of forgetting in my participants' discursive narration of filial piety.

It is important to briefly explain at this point that the term 'forgetting' does not necessarily indicate that there has been a proactive erasure of memories of the past. In the perspective of discourse analysis, forgetting does not literally mean to forget. As discussed in Chapter 4, there being a taboo about the GLF and CR does not mean that the Chinese government or the general public completely forbids talk of those periods. However, there is a strong tendency to avoid talking about the topic and to not mention aspects that might confuse or contradict currently preferred perceptions and sociopolitical trajectories.

This discourse of forgetting became noticeable when I began to subject comments, such as the following two statements, which were also presented in the previous chapter, to more critical analysis in light of historical events.

> P16: As children, we consider my mother did not have it easy raising us, especially in 'those years'. She also raised our children too. We feel that she has suffered a lot in her life. We need to step up and be filial to her now. (P16: a son, aged 51–60, married, mother was ill)
> P19: How do I put it . . . my father cannot do much work such as the heavy lifting and growing crops that he used to do. They have had many years of the hard life. You know how hard it was in those years. . . . As their son, I should do my part. I want them to rest for a few years. Maybe when he gets better, he can keep some chickens and ducks. I hope he can live a few years. (P19: a son, aged 41–50, married, father was ill)

As shown in P16 and P19's comments as well as explained in Chapter 7, in the participants' minds, their parents were figures who represented selflessness, sacrifice, and dedication. In order to repay the hardships and sacrifices of their parents, the participants needed to be filial. I asked them how much their parents had to suffer. Many of them gave me surprisingly similar explanations. As P5 (a daughter, aged 31–40, married, mother was ill) said, 'You know, being a farmer is quite hard, especially in those years. There was not much food or clothing'.

Despite the broadly perceived hardships due to a scarcity of material goods during the GLF and CR, P5 also expressed that being a farmer itself involves a life of hardship and sacrifice. This contrasts with the political depictions of farmers during the CR as noble and happy figures (Rofel, 2007). It seemed the participants were also not clear about, or forgot the details of, their parents' lives in those years. Did the narratives of sacrifice that replaced awareness of filial disobedience come from personal experience or collective memories, or did they result from a tragic national period, political manipulation, or all of these multilayered factors to form into the present discourse of filial piety? The participants imagined the lives of their parents to have contained nothing but selfless sacrifice and hardship in 'those years' (during the GLF and CR).

Forgetting Different Trajectories of Filial Piety

Another indication of the process of forgetting emerged when participants were asked if they thought there had been changes in the extent to which people adhered to filial piety in the present as compared to during different chronological stages in Chinese history. In response, most participants spoke as if filial piety was a static phenomenon that had persisted before economic reform for thousands of years. For example, P16 said, 'The past was all the same. People were always filial'. Below is another example demonstrating how participants had a tendency to treat the Mao era as part of an unchanging cultural continuum that had only begun to alter in recent times.

> P3: I think the social circumstances have changed. In the past, if someone were to not be filial or to abuse their parents, their affairs would be made public and punished in those years. Nowadays, only morality chastises those who are unfilial. It is less straightforward. In the past, people took care of their parents, talked to them, and were there with them. In the present, people are not with their parents. They only provide financial care. Nothing more. (P3: a son, aged 41–50 years old, married, father was ill)

P3 spoke as if people of his parents' generation practised filial piety in the same way that Chinese people had been practising it for the past 5,000 years. For P3, filial piety was a cultural norm that had not changed for the millennia. He tried to match his own personal experiences and perceptions up to a discursive formation of static filial piety. Of course, this static understanding is at odds with the fact that culture itself is dynamic and varies in different discursive situations (Song, 2008).

History is, as Foucault (1967) also suggested, non-linear. However, an understanding of tradition or a cultural norm as static is much easier for many people to grasp and might be a more useful tool for the purpose of achieving a certain discursive construction. It is not the case that filial piety has been the same continuously for several thousands of years. For example, it was highly criticised during the New Culture Movement (in the 1910s and 1920s) and the CR (Ikels, 2004). The discourse of forgetting was formed to obscure the constantly evolving nature of filial piety. It enables the period of the GLF and CR, and even the New Culture Movement, to blend into the constructed cultural continuum of filial piety, as long as these periods are understood and referred to in vague terms rather than exposed to detailed critique.

That Which Has Been Forgotten

After the New Culture Movement, and especially during the GLF and CR, filial piety was subjected to much ideological criticism (Poškaitė, 2014). Filial piety symbolised what feudalism (serfdom and the rule of nobility) stood for, namely the suppression of people's free minds, something unscientific and backward (Li, 2003; Xiao, 1999; Yu, 1996). People were encouraged to go against and abandon respect for their parents. It was a time during which the practice and perception of filial piety was overwhelmingly challenged by leading scholars, by the government, and subsequently by ordinary Chinese people (Ikels, 2006). Wang (2014) recounted a story of a son who reported his mother for her political opinions in 1970 during the CR and who subsequently had his mother sentenced to death for antirevolutionary beliefs. In 1980, the court overturned that verdict with a finding of not guilty.

Wang's (2014) story concerned an urban family, and as such it can be presumed to have been heavily influenced by political propaganda. Although peasant families could be argued to be under less pressure to denounce their parents, during my fieldwork in China, my mother told me a story about how my paternal grandfather, who came from a poor rural peasant family, responded positively to the government's call to rebel against his own father in those years. He was in his 20s at that time (during the 1950s and 1960s). My grandfather scolded his father in front of everyone in the village for being 'backward' and 'traditional' and burnt all of his father's ancient Chinese philosophy and fortune-telling books. Of course, this had been a taboo topic in our family, and I had not heard this story before. My mother told me this when she understood what I was trying to achieve for my Ph.D. research. She also asked me not to tell my father that I had heard this from her.[1] Perhaps she felt able to tell me this story because my paternal grandfather was not her own father, so she did not have to feel too guilty for revealing this family taboo topic. In the Chinese literature I have found similar accounts showing the extent to which much children disobeyed their parents and how severely

[1] Following suggestions from both of my supervisors, I asked my mother whether she would allow me to disclose the story in my thesis. She was made fully aware that her husband and father-in-law would potentially identify himself from the written story, although the likelihood is low since neither of them speak any English. My mother was highly supportive of my putting this story in the final thesis.

people and scholars criticised filial piety during the New Culture Movement, GLF, and CR (Ikels, 2006; Li, 2003; Xiao, 1999; Yu, 1996; Zang, 2000). Therefore, even children from poorer peasant families, who may have been less likely to denounce their parents compared to their urban counterparts, were for a time required to accept an ideology that put the Communist Revolution before family—an ideology that would have made them feel justified in denouncing their parents if it had proved necessary.

Another interesting example of how attitudes towards filial piety changed can be found in a newspaper article (*Dongfeng*, August 29 and September 1, 1966) notifying a change of name for Xiaogan city. The city changed its name to Dongfeng (eastern wind) because its former name, Xiaogan ('filial sense'), contained references to filial piety (Yu, 2002). The name Xiaogan came from a mythical story about a filial son receiving blessings in all aspects of his life in return for being filial (Yu, 2002). During the CR, the city's name change signalled the dismissal of traditional filial piety (Yu, 2002).

During the GLF and CR, the parents of my participants did not make sacrifices just for their families but, in a sense, more out of political conviction and as a political pursuit that many later came to see as having been hollow (Rofel, 2007). Children were encouraged by extreme leftist politicians and scholars to renounce their parents for the sake of eradicating Confucianism and other Chinese traditional ethics and philosophies (Yu, 1996; Zang, 2000). In some parts of China, parents were even treated violently and aggressively disobeyed (Ikels, 2004).

Interlinkage Between Forgetting and Parent Sacrifice

How did participants' parents practice filial piety during the CR? Many of the participants were not sure what happened or simply thought their parents were as filial as they were themselves. However, the literature contradicts this perception that filial piety was historically uniformly appreciated, identifying that filial piety was characterised as backward and feudal during the CR (Rofel, 2007). The history of 'those years' (as the GLF and CR are often collectively referred to) might willingly be forgotten, since under current filial discourse it is not considered 'decent' anymore to denounce filial piety. All participants, with the exception of one, had positive 'memories' about filial practice in the age of GLF and CR. One of the possible reasons for this might be that many participants were still quite young when these social criticisms of filial piety occurred, therefore may not be able to remember accurately. More likely, however, the forgetting discourse simplified the story into a version that worked for the presently required discourse that revalidates and values filial piety. Stories about the deprived material conditions during the GLF and CR were remembered and magnified to serve the same purpose; the extent to which filial piety was attacked was forgotten.

The discourse of forgetting was related to perceptions of parental sacrifice. Participants had to forget their parents' involvement in political pursuits and their criticism of filial piety in 'those years' to enable them to construct a discourse around their parents' hardship and sacrifice during the GLF and CR. A forgetting discourse, together with a parental sacrifice discourse, gave participants a reason to care at this critical time at the end of their parents' lives. In order to maintain filial piety against the challenges posed by the participants' social and economic circumstances, they needed to have a powerful perception of parental sacrifice and they needed to forget experiences or knowledge that contradicted this perception. Historical filial piety was purposefully (and also unconsciously or subconsciously) constructed through a forgetting mechanism. The alternative history of filial piety under attack in 'those years' remained hidden to a great extent. If stories of how filial piety was attacked during the CR were buried, the possibility of forming more complex understandings was also buried. This research aimed to investigate the complexity of filial discourse, and this can only be achieved by acknowledging the forgotten.

Forgetting for Different Generations

In this research, the youngest participant (P23) was 25 years old (the only participant in the 21–30 age group). Except for this one participant, whose parents were born right after the beginning of the CR, all other participants' parents had lived through almost all of the CR (1966–1976) and partially through the GLF (1958–1962) in their adult lives. Participants themselves were either very young children (too young to remember anything before the CR ended) or had not yet been born (the participant in her 20s and the other two participants in their early 30s).

As mentioned earlier, the CR and GLF are somewhat taboo topics for Chinese people, and this was reflected in the way participants often referred to it through the euphemism 'those years'. Even though participants did not talk about the CR explicitly, it appeared that they expected me to know what they meant by 'those years'. When P19 said in the quotation in the last section, 'You know how hard it was in those years', he assumed I knew about the hardship during the GLF and CR. This may suggest this hardship was a collective memory for Chinese people, at least for people born before me (I was born in 1986). P19, in his interview, suggested that it was a period of suffering, limited resources, hunger, and hardship, which contributed to the participants' perception of parental sacrifice in 'those years'.

Although naming the CR is politically taboo and the topic is perhaps too sensitive for many to say the words out loud, a small number of participants did explicitly use the words 'Cultural Revolution' in their interview, as shown in the example below. However, their association of the era with hardship and sacrifice is not particularly different from other participants.

> P7: Yes. Because material conditions are so too good now, they [the younger generation] don't know how the older generation lived. They have forgotten about many things. Our father's generation told us about things such as the Cultural Revolution, the people's commune system and what they suffered then.[2] (P7: a son, aged 41–50, married, father was ill)

As also explained by P7 (who was in his 40s), his parents' generation had told their children about how hard life was during the CR and during the time of the people's communes, such that his generation still knew about the trials their parents had endured back then. He also said that he, like many people in his generation (born in the 1960s and early 1970s), had also endured hardship when they were young children at the end of the CR and the beginning of economic reform. Therefore, he explained, they truly understood how hard it was for their parents and the need to repay them. However, he thought the younger generation (he mentioned 'your generation' as in my generation, which was born in the late 1980s) had forgotten about those harsh times.

For P7's generation, this forgetting might be different from that of the generation born in and after the 1980s. Considering P7's expressed beliefs, it appeared that his generation might have forgotten their parents'

[2] The people's commune system was the Soviet Union's way of establishing collective combinations of farm households where everyone worked together, sharing all the resources and outcomes. This served political, economic, and governmental functions (X. Chang, 2013) [not in reference list].

political pursuits and ideals, while, according to him, for the younger generation it was the hardship of 'those years' that was forgotten.

The generation that came after P7 has been far removed from any material hardship or scarcity of resources. P7 feared that this younger generation would therefore forget (he specifically used the word 'forget') about the hardships and sacrifices his parents' and his own generation made to raise their children. In order to maintain filiality for the younger generation, his generation might need to strengthen the parental sacrifice discourse enough for it to also influence their offspring. As a matter of fact, however, the younger generation, both P9 (in his early 30s) and P23 (in his 20s), expressed their appreciation for all the sacrifices their parents had made, even though they did not mention the CR, even obliquely (they were not yet born during the CR). They said that their parents 'suffered a lot when I was young' (P9: a son, aged 31–40, divorced, father was ill). Parental sacrifice discourse was indeed shown to have expanded into the younger generation in my research.

Participants' narratives showed that as they became parents themselves and grew older, they began to consider it necessary to impose a notion of parental sacrifice on their own children in order to encourage and maintain filial piety in the next generation. From the participants' accounts of their endeavours to make their children aware of this, perceptions of parental sacrifice not only emerged on the part of children but were also propelled by the parents' generation. Perceptions of parental sacrifice were not purely imagined and constructed by the children's generation due to their collective attempts to forget about a national, social, and political tragedy (Kleinman & Kleinman, 1994). These perceptions were also encouraged by their parents. This suggests that parental sacrifice and forgetting discourses are not specific to the current Chinese context. It is possible that these discourses have existed in the past as an important mechanism to sustain and transmit filial piety in Chinese society. This will be further discussed in Chapter 9.

Complexity of the Discursive Construction of Filial Piety by Different Generations

Many participants suggested that filial piety was not as strongly practised by the younger generation. For instance, P3 thought people provide more financial care than emotional care nowadays compared to in the past.

> P3: It is different. In the past, if your parents got sick, not only did you have to take care of them, you also needed to live with them. Nowadays, you can put them in a home and ask someone else to take care of them, if you have money of course. This way you fulfil your responsibilities, but you are not being filial. There is a difference here. A family bond is not about whether you give money or not. There are some older people who want to go into a home because they have friends there. If the older people don't want to go, their children will say to them, "You have to understand that I need to work". Many older people want to live with their children due to our traditional culture. This creates a distinction. In the past people paid attention to cultivating their relationships with parents or to strengthening their bonds. Nowadays people tend to use money to solve everything in this money-based society. The communication with parents has been reduced or is being paid less attention to. (P3: a son, aged 41–50 years old, married, father was ill)

P3's tone of voice conveyed that he thought this phenomenon, whereby people no longer provide their parents with direct care, to be a negative change. However, some participants actually thought filial practices had improved compared to previously. As suggested by P15 in the comment below, these participants thought the new generation understood filial piety better than the older generation because of its higher level of education.

> P15: The next generation will understand what filial piety is. However, our generation is a different story. Some of them don't understand it that much. They think filial piety is to provide financial assistance. However, filial piety never just means that . . . There are some changes. My generation doesn't have a hard and bitter life (*xinku*) as our parents did. And my daughter's generation is well educated [so his daughter can understand what filial piety really is]. (P15: a son, aged 41–50, married, mother was ill)

According to P15, his generation did not understand filial piety very well due to a lack of school-based education. P15 may also be an allusion to filial piety not being positively educated for or promoted during the CR, although he did not directly say this. His child's generation, born after the CR, did have the chance to be 'properly' educated about filial piety. He thinks these younger people are able to develop a more complex understanding of filial piety. P15 mentioned that material conditions had improved for his generation compared to his parents' generation (indicating that he still remembered the past as full of hardship and material deprivation for his parents.) This meant, firstly, that his daughter would be less guilt-driven in her relationship with him. Secondly, his daughter did not need to work as hard or as much as he had been working to provide the necessary financial care for his parents. Therefore, his daughter could focus on being filial to him in more ways than just the financial. Being filial might mean providing more emotional care or simply bonding with him.

P4 also deemed the present time to be a positive transition period for filial piety in terms of children being able to provide better care for their parents.

> P4: In the past, people were so poor. They tried to give as much as they could. In my generation, most people have at least a few thousand RMB [Chinese yuan]. People can send their ill parents to hospital for a cure. The big difference is money. Nowadays, we do have the ability to make our parents better. For example, my grandfather had blood hypertension. He died very early of that because my family did not have money to buy medicine back then. (P4: a daughter, aged 41–50, married, mother was ill)

P4 later also said that people nowadays received more education and were therefore more concerned about their parents' emotional needs, whereas in the past, people were more concerned about material conditions because there was not enough money to meet basic survival needs.

This difference between P4 and P3, in terms of their views about intergenerational filiality, does not necessarily reflect a contradiction, even though it seems as if they express completely opposite views from one another. The standard of emotional care and material care (financial care) varies for different people and in different scenarios. For P3, expressions of emotional care included living with one's parents and being there for them. He thought this has occurred less often over recent times because of the distance between parents and adult migrant peasant workers. P4 noted that compared to people before economic reforms, the younger generation in the rural areas now obtained much more education. Therefore, he explained, they would know how to talk to their parents and connect with them. This also relates to the point made in Chapter 7, that family members do not verbally state that they 'love' each other. Nevertheless, participants believed that the younger generation expressed their emotions more explicitly than the older generation.

Different layers of understanding of filial piety, including different historical understandings, demonstrate the complex nature of filial discourse and of how care might be expressed in actions, in being present, or in signs of empathy and understanding. The different views of P3 and the other two participants (P4 and P15) indicated both forgetting and remembering. As P3 forgot past criticisms of filial piety that had occurred at a national level, P4 and P15 started to remember something negative about the older generation in terms of filial practice compared to the present.

Complexity of Forgetting

Most participants did not reveal any negative views about filial practices during the GLF and CR when they were asked about the difference between the older and younger generation. As a matter of fact, one participant described filial piety as having been strongly adhered to during the CR:

> P3: In 'those years', people often talked about who is not filial. Public discourse supported this too. If someone was not filial, they would be publicly exposed for it. Those kinds of people were despised by everyone. It pushed people to fulfil their filial piety and it also stood as a warning for those people . . . People still condemn those who do not fulfil their filial responsibilities nowadays. However, it is not as straightforward as it was before. For example, when I was little, there was a guy who physically and verbally abused his parents. The village leader dragged him to the village square and condemned him with the support of all the villagers. He was also punished by having to pay for a movie for the village [which cost a lot for a peasant at that time]. This was a typical example. Nowadays, those [unfilial people] can only be condemned morally. Nobody actually comes to take care of this. (P3: a son, aged 41–50, married, father was ill)

For P3 during the CR, the public condemnation of unfilial practices was strong. Did he imagine it or did it really happen? According to Foucault (2012), history can be reinterpreted through the lens of current discourses. People's memory of the past is highly susceptible to the influence of present knowledge. However, one thing is certain from this participant's story: the discourse of filial piety is very complex. Even in accounts of the GLF and CR, there is not one simple truth or even perception of whether people were filial or not.

Political and Public Forgetting

Not only had participants forgotten the multiple realities of their parents' lives but the public also forgot its history of having once rebelled against filial piety during the GLF and CR. In recent years, the government has engaged in political discourse promoting Chinese traditional culture including filial piety and has set new laws such as the 2013 'parent-visiting law', under which if children do not visit their parents regularly they may be punished. Thus, the discourse of filial piety is also invoked for economic convenience to avoid an unsustainable welfare system.

The emergence, in recent years, of an increasingly dominant discourse of reviving filial piety requires a certain degree of forgetting. The required forgetting is not merely philosophical and individual but also political. There is no denying that filial piety entered a tremendously complicated and even chaotic period after it came under attack during the GLF and CR. Filial piety was further challenged by more recent structural changes, including economic and social changes, that resulted in changes to family structures and relationships. Eventually, these social consequences became sufficiently worrying that both the Chinese government and the Chinese people recognised a need for intervention. As part of this reckoning, to achieve a resolution to social disruption, lost stories may need to be retold in order to make sense of the complexity of filial piety in today's Chinese society.

Changing the Political Discourse of the 'Peasant'

The post-1978 modernisation project of the Chinese government has led to a cultivation of the perception that being a peasant results in hardship (as opposed to material comfort and development), as a way of legitimating and promoting the economic reforms (Kipnis, 2007; Rofel, 2007). In order to attain a 'modern' life, peasants have to go to the big cities to work and support their families (Lin, 2013). As discussed in Chapter 2, migrant peasant workers are disadvantaged by urban public policies compared to their urban counterparts. P15 expressed his marginalised social status:

> P15: I feel like I did not offer them enough care before. I have this guilt inside of me that tortures me, even though I often phone them and ask them not to do any farm work. And if they need money, I will send some to them. You see, my wife's parents are over 80, and mine are over 70. And we can't earn much money outside [in the big city] given our poor educational background. The urban residents of Guangdong often earn much more than us migrant workers from other provinces. The salary for a junior manager is normally 5,000 RMB [per month]. It is much less for ordinary workers. My child's college education costs 30,000 RMB per year. This means there is only a little bit left that I can provide for my parents. (P15: a son, aged 41–50, married, mother was ill)

For P15, working in the big city was a necessity because he needed to support his parents who were over 70 and his parents-in-law who were over 80-years old. Moreover, it is commonly understood that working in big cities is a meaningful social practice, even if workers are socially marginalised. Urbanisation is seen as positive progress, as promoted by the modernisation project (Rofel, 2007). Not being able to bring his parents to the city in which he and his wife were working and not being able to live together with his parents left P15 feeling guilty. This comment and the guilt and regret reflected in it also relate to the discourse about parental sacrifice, because P15's parents missed out on the wonderful things that living in the city supposedly provided access to.

Current research on Chinese migrant peasant workers tends to focus on their vulnerable or marginalised social status, especially by comparison to their bourgeois urban counterparts (Lin, 2013). Many scholars (Guan, 2005; Lin, 2013; Rofel, 2007) have suggested that recent literature tends to identify migrant peasant workers as a group with problems and not 'modern'. According to Shi (2009), a traditional perception of filial piety is still strong in rural China where ancestral beliefs still have some degree of influence, compared to in urban areas. Lin (2013) identified this strong sense of filiality, as associated with the discourse of migrant peasant workers not being 'modern'. This assumption has positioned traditional culture as in opposition to a 'modern' identity and a big-city lifestyle (Lin, 2013). Rofel (2007) claimed the 'modernisation project' carried out by the Chinese government and society has propelled the construction of rural areas, migrant peasant worker lifestyles, and related traditional culture as not modern. However, as Whyte and Ikels (2004) have pointed out, fulfilling filial responsibilities in rural areas may be motivated more by practicality than by adherence to cultural beliefs; rural Chinese have no option but to rely on traditional family systems of support because they receive insufficient social welfare assistance. Nonetheless, the public perception of migrant peasant workers as being not modern carries biased connotations of backwardness and dysfunctionality.

This taken for granted categorisation of migrant peasant workers as vulnerable and marginalised overlooks that the 'peasant' was once a heroic figure during the GLF and CR. Peasants were politically promoted as heroic and upright, while capitalists and landlords were depicted as evil and backward (Mou et al., 2013). However, since economic reform 'peasant' has gradually become a term of disdain, associated with being unfashionable, poor, and not 'modern' (Mou et al., 2013). In today's political and public discourse, the 'peasant' is not a heroic figure.

'Parent-Visiting Law': Law Versus Morality

On July 1, 2013, a new law came into effect in China legally obliging adult children to visit parents. According to the law, adult children who fail to comply with visiting requirements can be sued by their parents and may face legal charges and punishment (Fan, 2013). Although there is recognition of the law's good intentions in terms of the revival of traditional virtue and morals, it has attracted some criticism, both domestically and internationally. More than half of the participants had heard of the law by the time of their interview with me (between November 2013 and April 2014). For those who had not heard of it, I provided an explanation. Most of the participants initially said that they thought the 'parent-visiting law' was 'effective', meaning that they thought it to be a positive thing. However, when I asked them whether the law had any impact on them, they answered no; even so, they said they supported it as a positive moral symbol. P1 commented on this law:

> I: What do you think about the new 'parent-visiting law'? Do you think it is effective?
> P1: Yes, I have heard of it. I think it is effective.
> I: Does it affect your caregiving for your parent?
> P1: No.
> I: Then why do you think it is effective?
> P1: Fulfilling filial responsibilities is a good tradition for Chinese people. Most of our people have fulfilled theirs.

> I: Since we already have this tradition that everyone follows, why do we need this law?
> P1: There are still a few people who don't fulfil their filial responsibilities. I am not sure about how this will affect those people. However, I think if there is a law to make it compulsory, then children have to follow it to some degree. Otherwise, they will be morally condemned.
> I: How do you think public morality and laws differ in terms of their effects?
> P1: A law will be enforceable, requiring people to do it. (P1: a daughter, aged 41–50, re-married, father was ill)

P1 was a daughter in her 40s who worked for the local government. She had been a migrant peasant worker for many years before her current profession. She had come back to work for the Langzhong local government a few years earlier through her connections with a relative. Her words carried several implications. First of all, she considered this law to be a positive social intervention. Morally, the introduction of the law was accepted and supported by her. She thought it served as a warning call for unfilial people to be filial. This demonstrates that the traditional value of filial piety as *Tianjingdiyi* remains embedded in Chinese people's cultural and emotional consciousness.

Dating back to ancient times and until the GLF and CR, there were many laws aimed at forcing people to be filial, including some requiring children to provide for elderly parents and others stipulating there should be three years of mourning for dead parents. During the GLF and CR, these ancient filial laws were criticised as exploitative of children. However, P1 now welcomed laws imposing filial practice for moral reasons. This participant's comment reflected the restoration of filial piety as a moral position that must be accepted and practised in China, although views on how this should be carried out in practice might differ or be negotiable.

It is important, with respect to analysing the interview data, to understand that there were contextual constraints to how participants could express themselves. Not supporting the law might be seen as unfilial. Therefore, participants might not be willing to openly express their true opinions about the law out of fear about what the interviewer might think of them if they did. A quote from P2 confirmed that participants might be concerned about being seen as inappropriately expressing uneducated opinions.

I: What do you think about the new 'parent-visiting law'?
P2: I have heard of it on TV.
I: Do you think it's effective?
P2: I think it is effective, because it is a law. However, from what I saw in a few television programmes, some family disputes would not be able to be resolved by official mediation. Therefore, it might not be as useful as it sounds.
I: Does it affect your caregiving for your parent?
P2: No, I just do what I am supposed to do as a child.
I: Then why do you think it's effective, since it won't affect your behaviour?
P2: I don't know. I am only a peasant; I don't know how to evaluate this. But I think if it's a law, there must be something good about it. (P2: a daughter, aged 31–40, married, father was ill)

The peasant workers who were participants in my interviews still tended to have a high level of respect for or fear around the law. Generally, the participants believed there must be a reason why the government instituted particular laws.

P1 stressed the importance of using education and propaganda to implement the law, as opposed to encouraging parents to sue their children.

I: In what way do you think the law should implement filial piety?
P1: Through education I think. I think soft measures such as education or propaganda should be implemented to achieve the goal.
I: Do you think parents would sue their children if they are unfilial?
P1: There are some who would, but not many. Although there are barely any parents who would actually accuse their children, I do think this law acts as a warning for those children who have been neglecting their parents.

A historical discourse that appeared to be reflected in the participants' commentaries is a Confucian understanding of law, which holds that a law's purpose is first to educate and only afterwards to enforce (Onsman, 2012). In Confucian ideology, implementing a law without also teaching and guiding people on how to obey the law is no different from setting a trap for them (Bell & Ham, 2003). P1's mention of 'soft measures' may indicate that she perceives filial piety more as a moral issue than a legal one. In her opinion, this law should provide incentives instead of punishment to encourage people to be filial.

There is an old saying in China that goes, 'Even the most virtuous government officials cannot resolve family matters'. Indeed, there are technical difficulties for officials attempting to resolve family disputes. In a familial relationship, it is often impossible to distinguish right from wrong or good from bad in the majority of cases. This makes it technically complicated for governmental institutions to enforce laws. For example, if unfilial children are sentenced to prison, who would be left to support their elderly parents? Would the government or civil society step in? As discussed in Chapter 2, China has not (yet) created a comprehensive social safety net for older persons. They may thus end up without any support. Thus, the law's implementation is problematic.

Despite their expressed reservations, however, participants' commentaries indicated that these migrant workers still had respect for, or perhaps feared, this particular law. Perhaps the 'parent-visiting law' will provide a reminder to Chinese people to be filial, as part of a larger project to return filial practice to mainstream discourse. If people believe the government has good intentions in introducing this law, the law will project an educational and strengthening purpose to some degree. There were two participants, quoted below, who felt strongly positive about the educational purpose of this law.

> I: Why do you think the government issued this law?
> P6: Nowadays young people go away to work, leaving their elders and children at home. They wouldn't even know if their parents got sick. This law monitors and pushes young people to visit their parents. (P6: a son, aged 31–40, married, father was ill)
> I: Have you heard of the 'parent-visiting law' issued this year?
> P4: Yes.
> I: Do you think it is effective?
> P4: It could manage and control [people's unfilial behaviours]. The generation born in the 1960s or 1970s have a strong responsibility towards their parents. The ones [born] after that might not be as responsible. For them, parents devote all they have to their children. The parents will give the children whatever they want. If they don't, in the end they will become 'criminals' to their children. This is my personal perspective. I am not sure how you young people think about this. There are only one or two children nowadays. They have received different treatment from birth. I don't think they would do what I do to care for my mother.
> I: Do you think this law has influenced you in any way?

P4: No. I know how I should treat my parents. Why would I need this law? (P4: a daughter, aged 41–50, married, mother was ill)

P4 did not have much faith in the future generation in terms of filial practice. She hoped the law would have an effect on that generation to make it more filial. This concern was echoed in a conversation I had with my grandfather during my fieldwork in which he expressed a similar worry to me. He asked me if I would be prepared to marry a woman (any woman) from my hometown city. At first I thought he might wish me to do this because he did not like the idea of having a granddaughter-in-law with a background that was too different from my own. However, as he later told me, he was worried about my parents' future. If one marries someone who comes from far away, inevitably one will have less time to spare to visit parents and parents-in-law because of the distances involved. My grandfather worried that my parents would see me less often. He said, 'I have three children who live in the same city as I do, but your parents only have you. If they become sick in the future, who will take care of them?' These worries about the situation of people with children born in the 1980s and 1990s facilitated participants' support for the law, to a great extent.

A story told by a participant who was born in the 1980s resonated with my grandfather's concerns. P9 strongly supported the 'parent-visiting law'. He was in his early 30s (born in the early 1980s) and was an only child. He worked as a construction contractor leading a group of builders in a big city within his home province (approximately four hours by bus from his hometown).

I: Why do you feel it is effective?

P9: There was a performance in one of the Spring Festival banquets talking about how none of the children of an old lady came back home when she had prepared a lot of food for the Spring Festival. I was moved by that scene.

I: From your story, does this mean this law has a warning effect?

P9: Yes, it has this effect.

I: Because you said it doesn't affect you, who do you think it would affect?

P9: I think it reminds people who are not filial about our traditional values and morality. It is hard now for both parents and children because most families only have one child. Before, if this child couldn't go back, the others would. It's different now since there is only one child. People will have time if they try to make some.

> I: In current Chinese society, there are many who go outside [their hometown] to work.
> P9: Many live outside too.
> I: They often have little time and money to visit their parents in the hometown. So you think they should take the time to visit more?
> P9: They can, they can.
> I: So you think this is not dependent on society or the government but on the children themselves?
> P9: Themselves. For example, nowadays, after men marry outside [their hometown], there are many reasons why his wife doesn't get along with his mother. You could find any reason. However, you can always squeeze in time, even when you are busy. (P9: a son, aged 31–40, divorced, father was ill)

P9 thought that no matter how busy or poor, one could always find a way to visit one's parents. His statements first signalled that he was filial without a doubt. Secondly, he supported the law because he did not have sympathy towards those who claimed to have difficulties in visiting home regularly. He thought that for most migrant peasant workers, claims about limited time and problematic financial situations were just excuses. Even after I gave some examples suggesting that some people might struggle, he repeated twice that 'they can [visit]'. Aware that some people born in the 1960s and 1970s held a negative view of those born in 1980s and 1990s in terms of the prevalence of filial practice, he felt proud of being filial and strongly supported the filial law. For P9, it was children's primary responsibility to visit and take care of their parents under any circumstances. It might be partially because of his own financial privilege and closer proximity to his parents compared to other participants (who all worked in cities in other provinces) that he seemed unable to empathise with others' difficulties. In any case, he supported the law in terms of its moral and educational guidance for people.

Lack of Workability and Usefulness of the 'Parent-Visiting Law'

By contrast to the expressed opinion on the 'parent-visiting law' of most of the participants (which might or might not have been their actual views as they may have been concerned with presenting themselves in a good light), the 'parent-visiting law' has been heavily criticised in the academic literature for its lack of workability (Fan, 2013). According to Park (2015), Korea, which is a country with a prominent Confucian cultural heritage, also resorted to legislation by instituting an Act on the Encouragement and Support of Filial Piety (in 2008). Park (2015, p. 280) noted that 'the nature of the law is largely rhetorical and symbolic rather than practical, and as a result, its workability and efficiency are limited'. Next follows an exploration of some of the reasons participants and academics have cast doubt on the workability of the Chinese 'parent-visiting law'.

Few Parents Would Sue Their Children. Few parents would report and sue their children for elder abuse and neglect (Chang et al., 2016; Dong et al., 2008), let alone for not visiting enough. As Ikels (2004) stated in her book *Filial Piety: Practice and Discourse in Contemporary East Asia*, Chinese parents are still strongly attached to the narrative of 'ugly business stays in the family'. Chinese people have a tendency to be highly protective of their family's 'face' or reputation (Ikels, 2004). This view was expressed by several participants.

> P16: Yes, I have heard [about the law]. However, there are no people in rural areas who would sue their children, because nobody knows how. There might be some in the urban areas.
> I: You think about 30% of rural Chinese people are not filial. Do you think their parents would sue them if they knew about the law?
> P16: Still no. They would be considerate for the sake of their children, especially the rural parents. (P6: a son, aged 31–40, married, father was ill)

According to P16 above, not many parents would sue their children. P16 mentioned that rural parents are less likely to sue their children compared to urban parents. There might be several reasons for this. One might be that rural residents adhere to more traditional cultural beliefs and practices and rural older persons have much less social security compared to older persons in urban areas. Another reason, suggested by P16, was that nobody in the rural areas knows how to sue, even if they have heard of the law through television or some other source. Urban residents were considered better educated and informed. In a way, rural parents are disempowered through a lack of knowledge. They are also disempowered by their less privileged material condition compared to their urban counterparts (Dai, 2015). As mentioned before, if they sue their children, on whom they depend, who will take care of them (Dai, 2015)?

No Consideration for Different Situations and No Specific Criteria for Enforcement. Three participants outright challenged the effectiveness and workability of the law. P3 was an only son with one sister, P21 was an only child (son), and P2 was an only child (daughter). All three participants commented that the law was not effective.

> P3: It doesn't sound that effective. It might be a little bit, but not so much. The government introduces this law, but who actually monitors it? Moreover, parents would think of their children. Even if their children hadn't visited them, they would lie for their children. There are some who sue their children for not visiting. However, most parents would stand with their children. The children might say, "You embarrassed me and my work will be negatively affected." I think this law needs to be reviewed. I doubt that it's effective.
> I: Why do you think the government made this law?
> P3: Because members of the Chinese People's Political Consultative Conference proposed it. I think it contains more symbolic than actual meaning. It is like an advertisement. You don't know how it will turn out.
> I: Has this law influenced the way you take care of your parents?
> P3: No. Nothing changed in my routine after this law came into effect. I work and I go back home for festivals and on holidays. When I am free, I go back. If not, I stay away. And I often call my parents to tell them that I am safe. Nothing actually changes [due to this law]. (P3: a son, aged 41–50 years old, married, father was ill)

P3 doubted the law's workability for two reasons. Firstly, there is no monitoring of adherence to it. Which institution will monitor how many times children visit their parents per year? How many times is enough? This would be situation-dependent. If migrant workers work in a remote area, it is much more difficult for them to visit compared to people who live and work closer to their parents. Secondly, few people would sue their own children. For P3, although it was a law, it was more like a political piece of propaganda and a moral framework.

If the point of the law is not to deliver actual punishment but rather to encourage filial practice among the public, then the law is likely to fail in its intentions unless it considers workability and the varying conditions people find themselves in, especially the one-child generation. P21 expressed the view that it is better to encourage people through an appeal to their values and good intentions than to try to enforce compliance by threatening them. To provide encouragement may require more government incentives as well as social support to create an environment supportive of caring for parents in need.

P23 considered it was 'sad' to attempt to enforce morality by law. If it was necessary to have a law to enforce filial piety, what does that say about how much filial practice and perception have diminished? P23 expressed his concern and regret about this change:

> I: Have you heard of the 'parent-visiting law' passed last year?
> P23: It could have a warning effect in terms of pushing people who don't visit their parents that often. However, it is quite sad and ineffective to use cold legislation to fix filial piety. (P23: a daughter, aged 21–30, single, mother was ill)

Conclusion

This chapter's main focus has been to explain how the discourse of filial piety can be understood through the discursive mechanism of forgetting. It is essential to understand that the public discourse of filial piety is different from the migrant peasant workers' subjective construction of filiality. Yet, these constructs are connected under the discourse of forgetting and involve various imaginings of the past (especially with respect to events during the CR). On the one hand, the government's leading role in promoting the ideology of filial piety might have positive effects on people's reconstruction of filial discourse (Ouyang & Cui, 2013). On the other hand, the government is still working on providing sufficient support for eldercare (James, 2002).

Migrant peasant workers are not merely a disadvantaged social group within the modernisation project. They are capable of making sense of themselves in the so-called modern world in the current Chinese context (Lin, 2013). According to He and van Heugten (2020), filial perceptions and familial values are major aspects of the identity migrant peasant workers construct for themselves. For my participants, subjective filial perception came from and depended on filial forgetting, which also interacted with public forgetting. It counteracted the public forgetting by highlighting a sense of parental sacrifice. The parental sacrifice not only involved imagined pasts (during the GLF and CR) but also the present (e.g., grandparenthood) as well as the future (the generational differences participants identified and thought needed attention through education and example setting). On the other hand, subjective filial piety acted to encourage participants to help themselves. In this research, participants provided care for their parents in need. However, filial discourses and practices also prevented people from asking or demanding help from the government and society.

Not only my participants but also the public seems to have forgotten or overlooked this contradiction and has thus far ignored the need to initiate an open dialogue about the conflicts in these policies and directions. Such dialogue would raise questions about the conflicts between modernisation and Chinese tradition and between western and Chinese philosophy. In the next chapter, I will engage in a deeper analysis and discussion of parental sacrifice and forgetting discourses, and also consider the epistemological location of the complexities and contradictions within the current filial discourse. Two different culture and philosophy clashes stand out in relation to this exploration: western modernity versus traditional Chinese culture, and Foucauldian discourse analysis versus Chinese philosophy. These clashes emerged in the research data and constantly shaped my methodological reflexivity.

References

Bell, D., & Ham, C. B. (2003). *Confucianism for the modern world*. Cambridge University Press.

Chang, F., Shi, Y., Yi, H., & Johnson, N. (2016). Adult child migration and elderly parental health in rural China. *China Agricultural Economic Review, 8*(4), 677–697. https://doi.org/10.1108/CAER-11-2015-0169

Dai, B. (2015). The old age health security in rural China: Where to go? *International Journal for Equity in Health, 14*(119), 1–6. https://doi.org/10.1186/s12939-015-0224-5

Dong, X., Simon, M. A., Odwazny, R., & Gorbien, M. (2008). Depression and elder abuse and neglect among a community-dwelling Chinese elderly population. *Journal of Elder Abuse & Neglect, 20*(1), 25–41. https://doi.org/10.1300/J084v20n01_02

Fan, F. (2013, July 2). Parent-visiting services offered in wake of law. *People*. Retrieved from http://en.people.cn

Foucault, M. (1967). *Madness and civilization: A history of insanity in the age of reason*. Tavistock.

Foucault, M. (1972). The confession of the flesh. In C. Gordon (Ed.), *Power/knowledge: Selected interviews and other writings 1972–1977* (pp. 194–228). Pantheon.

Foucault, M. (2000). The subject and power. In J. D. Faubion (Ed.). The New Press.

Foucault, M. (2012). *The history of sexuality (vol. 2). The use of pleasure*. Vintage.

Guan, Y. (2005). Legal protection for traditional knowledge and traditional culture expressions '传统知识及传统文化表达的法律保护问题'. *Normal University of Guizhou University Press (Social Science), 2*(3), 14–26.

He, L., & van Heugten, K. (2020). Chinese migrant workers' care experiences: A model of the mediating roles of filial piety. *Qualitative Health Research, 30*(11), 1–13. https://doi.org/10.1177/1049732320925420

Ikels, C. (2004). *Filial piety: Practice and discourse in contemporary East Asia*. Stanford University Press.

Ikels, C. (2006). Economic reform and intergenerational relationships in China. *Oxford Development Studies, 34*(4), 387–400. https://doi.org/10.1080/13600810601045619

James, E. (2002). How can China solve its old-age security problem? The interaction between pension, state enterprise and financial market reform. *Journal of Pension Economics and Finance, 1*(1), 53–75. https://doi.org/10.1017/S1474747202001026

Kipnis, A. (2007). Neoliberalism reified: Suzhi discourse and tropes of neoliberalism in the People's Republic of China. *Journal of the Royal Anthropological Institute, 13*(2), 383–400. https://doi.org/10.1111/j.1467-9655.2007.00432.x

Kleinman, A., & Kleinman, J. (1994). How bodies remember: Social memory and bodily experience of criticism, resistance, and delegitimation following China's Cultural Revolution. *New Literary History, 25*(3), 707–723. https://doi.org/10.2307/469474

Li, G. (2003). Luxun's critique over feudal filial piety during the May Fourth Movement 五四时期鲁迅对封建孝道的批判. *Huxiang Forum 湖湘论坛* (2), 85–85. http://hxlt.xueshu.com/

Lin, X. (2013). *Gender, modernity and male migrant workers in China: Becoming a 'modern' man*. Routledge.

Mou, J., Griffiths, S. M., Fong, H., & Dawes, M. G. (2013). Health of China's rural–urban migrants and their families: A review of literature from 2000 to 2012. *British Medical Bulletin, 106*(1), 19–43. https://doi.org/10.1093/bmb/ldt016

Onsman, A. (2012). Recognising the ordinances of Heaven: The role of Confucianism in higher education management in the People's Republic of China. *Journal of Higher Education Policy and Management, 34*(2), 169–184. https://doi.org/10.1080/1360080X.2012.662741

Ouyang, J., & Cui, C. (2013). The cultivation of Chinese traditional culture and socialist core value perceptions '中国传统文化与社会主义核心价值观的培育'. *Shandong Social Science 山东社会科学, 3*, 11–15. http://www.sdshkx.com/

Park, H. (2015). Legislating for filial piety: An indirect approach to promoting family support and responsibility for older people in Korea. *Journal of Aging & Social Policy, 27*(3), 280–293. https://doi.org/10.1080/08959420.2015.1024536

Poškaitė, L. (2014). Filial piety (*xiao* 孝) for the contemporary and global world. *Asian Studies, 2*(1), 99–114. https://doi.org/10.4312/as.2014.2.1.99-114

Rofel, L. (2007). *Desiring China: Experiments in neoliberalism, sexuality, and public culture*. Duke University Press.

Shi, L. (2009). 'Little quilted vests to warm parents' hearts': Redefining the gendered practice of filial piety in rural north-eastern China. *The China Quarterly, 198*(198), 348–363. https://doi.org/10.1017/S0305741009000344

Song, Z. (2008). *Chinese traditional philosophical discussion 中国传统哲学通*. People's University of China Press.

Wang, Y. (2014). *Chinese traditional filial piety and contemporary rural family elder care research 中国传统孝道思想与当代农村家庭养老研究*. QingHai Normal University 青海师范大学.

Whyte, M. K., & Ikels, C. (2004). Filial obligations in Chinese families: Paradoxes of modernization. In C. Ikels (Ed.), *Filial piety: Practice and discourse in contemporary East Asia*. Stanford University Press.

Xiao, Q. (1999). A discussion of the critique of traditional filial piety in the May Fourth period 五四时期对传统孝道的批判. *Lanzhou Transportation University Press 兰州交通大学学报* (4), 38–43. http://xb.lzjtu.edu.cn/CN/volumn/home.shtml

Yu, X. (2002). 'Xiaogan' renamed to 'Dongfeng' during the Cultural Revolution 文革" 中 "孝感" 改名叫 "东风. *China Geography: Administration Area and Place Name 中国方域: 行政区划与地名, 6*, 38–38.

Yu, Y. (1996). Criticism and reconstruction of traditional filial piety in recent history 近代中国知识分子对传统孝道的批判与重建. *Dongyueluncong 东岳论丛* (2), 77–82. http://www.sdass.net.cn/Info/?id=86

Zang, X. (2000). *Children of the cultural revolution: Family life and political behavior in Mao's China*. Westview.

CHAPTER 9

Migrant Peasant Workers' Care Experiences in Relation to the Three Conceptual Similarities Between Foucauldian and Chinese Philosophies

Introduction

My research started out by asking a seemingly broad research question: how do Chinese migrant workers make sense of caring for parents with cancer? I quickly discovered that they did so through discourses of filial piety, and that filial piety plays a complicated mediating role in participants' care experiences. Two main discourses emerged from the data analysis: a parental sacrifice discourse and a forgetting discourse (public forgetting and filial forgetting). These two discourses had a discursive focus on the Great Leap Forward (GLF) and the Cultural Revolution (CR). The analysis identified how participants used parental sacrifice and forgetting discourses to make sense of their caring roles and construct their filial selves. The concept of filiality is both complex and relational. Participants' discursive constructions of their care experiences also reflected a strong orientation towards action/practice.

The second research question asked how Chinese migrant workers are affected by changes in discourses of filial piety in current Chinese society. In exploring this question, I considered contextual changes synthesised from the literature on filial practices and theories and research participants' explanations of the changes in filial piety they had experienced

L. He, *Care Work, Migrant Peasant Families and Discourse of Filial Piety in China*, https://doi.org/10.1007/978-981-16-1880-2_9

and perceived. In their discussions, participants contrasted their perceptions of filial piety in the past, the present, and the future and expressed their worry that the next generation would be less filial than they were. The discourse of parental sacrifice that unfolded may be specific to the generation of my participants, due to the strong connection of this cohort to the GLF and the CR. Filial piety, as practised by the participants in this research, may not necessarily be able to be practised in the same way by future generations of rural workers. However, a closer examination, including of the literature, shows that the parental sacrifice discourse that supported participants' maintenance of filial piety is not a new phenomenon. And with respect to the future, several of the youngest participants had also adopted the idea of parental sacrifice.

In the next section, I will consider how this research might contribute to resolve the unsettling questions that surround the concept of the continuing place of filial piety in Chinese society at the present time, and into the future. Based on the findings of my research, the first step in reconciling conflicted ideas and ideals of filial piety starts with remembering the purposeful denigration of filial piety and lack of respect for elders that was promoted during the GLF and CR (Xiao, 2001). Understanding the discursive construction of parental sacrifice and forgetting discourses elicits the possibility that filial piety might be strengthened through supporting these two mechanisms of participants' filial construction with new, previously obscured, content and information. This is particularly important for future generations.

When people start to remember, they may gain the capacity for parrhesia ('to speak candidly or to ask forgiveness for so speaking'; Foucault, 1999, p. 5) in relation to matters that have been taboo. The other potential usefulness of this rhetorical technique drawn from Foucault includes its appropriateness in relation to engaging in theorising for practice in human services; this is also discussed in this chapter.

The First Research Question: How Do Chinese Migrant Workers Make Sense of Caring for Parents with Cancer?

When I asked participants why they came back to care for their parents, they all said it was a duty. Every one of them talked about filial piety being important for Chinese people. When I sought to understand how participants made sense of caring for parents diagnosed with cancer, the importance of filial piety quickly became apparent.

It is not hard to see how contextual changes such as urbanisation and governmental policies such as the one-child policy have presented difficult challenges for migrant peasant workers in their efforts to fulfil their filial responsibilities. Some filial caregiving behaviours have been altered in these recent major social transformation processes. For instance, the main caregiver used to be the eldest daughter-in-law in ancient Chinese society. In my research, from observations in fieldwork and as reflected in participants' stories, sons and daughters now appeared to be the main source of hands-on caregivers.

Participants resorted to discursive mechanisms to make sense of their present filial caring experiences and to enable them to confront the challenges posed by contextual modernisation-related changes. From analysing participants' interviews, two main discourses surfaced: a parental sacrifice discourse and a forgetting discourse. As shown in the previous two chapters, these two discourses were important mechanisms or processes through which participants negotiated their ability to remain filial and engage in the care of their parents despite the challenges they faced.

A Discursive Focus on the Period of the GLF and the CR

According to Halperin (1998), it is easy to forget recent history. This may be so because it is difficult for people to stand back from recent events in which they or their loved ones have participated. Seeing more clearly may have relational repercussions. From most of the participants' perspectives, filial piety had only changed after economic reforms that commenced in 1978. However, it is known that the discourse of filial piety in fact continuously evolved over 2,000 years. The forgetting discourse identified in this research was not a simple matter of merely glossing over complexities and generalising about historical events for ease of explanation: it involved a more deeply embedded structural forgetting.

Foucault claimed that history is abrupt instead of linear (Foucault, 1970). I suggest that perhaps forgetting facilitates the accommodation of abrupt, discontinuous, and non-linear features of history. When a fraction of recent history is forgotten, that historical fraction becomes broken and disrupted and is no longer 'lineal'.

The Complexity of Filial Discourse in the Chinese Context. The findings of my research show that the claim that neoliberalism diminished filial practice in contemporary Chinese society is too simplistic. This claim arises in the literature in association with the assumption that Chinese society has gradually become neoliberal over recent decades following the 1978 economic reforms. The belief that neoliberalism exerts a negative influence on filial practice has raised questions about the impact of neoliberalism on current Chinese society. The recent 'modernisation project' comprised a series of neoliberal tendencies such as marketisation (Wu, 2010). Additionally, the promotion of cultural filial piety that has been pursued in the public discourse in recent years suggests an inclination to avoid building a more comprehensive welfare system. This public discourse shows neoliberal traits of retreat from responsibilities. Therefore, some scholars have claimed that China has fully embraced neoliberalism (Anagnost, 2004; Greenhalgh & Winckler, 2005; Hairong, 2003). However, many other refuted such a claim by claiming it is much more complex in China (Kipnis, 2007; Ma, 2009).

As my research has shown, Chinese society is complex and, while an easy scapegoat, neoliberalism is not the sole cause of a decline in filial practice. The critique and denigration of filial piety that took place during the GLF and CR, for example, should also bear the blame for this decline. The simplistic claim that neoliberalism is the root cause of a diminishment of filial practice is in part due to the silence surrounding the GLF and CR, as part of a complex forgetting discourse that has involved both the government and the Chinese people.

Public Forgetting, Filial Forgetting, and Parental Sacrifice. The discourse of public forgetting comes with a series of self-contradictions. Past political, scholarly, and publicly espoused ideologies and actions are reconstructed in the form of a more morally acceptable discourse of hardship and sacrifice, because many of those past motivations do not have legitimacy in the present (Forkel & Silbereisen, 2001). The current status of migrant peasant workers stands in contradiction to the political discourse during 'those years' that presented the peasant as a hero figure (Lin, 2013; Mou et al., 2013). The political and public discourse appears to have forgotten its glorification of the peasant class and its heavy criticism of filial piety during the GLF and CR. The Chinese government has been promoting filial piety through policies such as the 'parent-visiting law' and appears to have forgotten its heavy criticism of filial piety during the GLF and CR (Wang, 2014; Xiao, 2001).

Participants' personal filial forgetting was interlinked and intertwined with public forgetting. As participants forgot about things such as the political pursuits of their parents during the GLF and CR, they also constructed a historical period of total parental sacrifice and hardship. Hardships that were depicted to have been endured by participants' parents during the GLF and CR were connected to a theme of 'not eating well' and 'not dressing well'. These hardships symbolised parental sacrifice, that is, a period of time filled with hardship and sacrifice with respect to raising their children.

During the GLF and CR, people, especially young people, were encouraged to consider themselves protectors of Communism (Rofel, 2007). This quickly turned into an uncontrolled populist power game including destructive activities (e.g., destroying cultural symbols and heritage) and fights (Wong, 1988). People fought each other thinking they were the true defenders of the Communist ideology and of the nation (Rofel, 2007). Parents were rebelled against by their children, and filial piety was heavily criticised by academic scholars and political journalists (Yan, 1999). The participants' stories about 'those years' emphasised a lack of food and clothing and of access to medical equipment and care, but not the other things stated above.

Even though the new generation born after CR was consistently told how hard life was when their parents' generation was growing up, the actual events of the GLF and CR remained a taboo topic. In the mainstream media, the GLF and CR are hardly discussed (Rofel, 2007). As noted, my participants used 'those years' as a substitute term for the GLF and CR, just as television programmes like *Ke Wang* 渴望 (Desire) did for this time period, according to Rofel (2007). Fears about speaking more openly are real.

The public forgetting discourse constitutes a particular way of exercising power rather than the direct overt ownership of a power over the public (Foucault, 2000). The public forgetting discourse interacted with the participants' forgetting in a complex way. There is a will on the part of both the government and the public to forget this tragic period. There is no doubt the Chinese governmental discourse plays a crucially important role in (re)constructing the current filial discourse, even though it is not the only force. Foucauldian discourse analyst Niels Andersen (2003) identified that governments play an important role in creating a sense of community and in helping shape people's public and private identities. Governments are only one of the foremost discursive forces, and these forces are further transmitted through various social institutions. Andersen's (2003) discursive analytical focus on institutional power is in line with Foucault's (1991) governmentality argument, and being conscious of Andersen's (2003) theorising and the theory of governmentality helped further my analysis of the Chinese government's involvement in the construction of filial discourse.

Scar Literature, Yiku Sitian, Parental Sacrifice, and Forgetting. Participants' narratives of parental sacrifice relate to what is dubbed 'scar literature伤痕文学' (Galik, 1982; Rofel, 2007). The story of the CR, when it is told, can also be considered to fit in with scar literature. In scar literature, which includes film as well as writing, parent generations are often portrayed as the victims of larger forces (Lee & Dutrait, 2001). They are seen as a generation ruined by meaningless power games that were engaged in by the powerful elite, from the top-down. The post-CR government broadly supported this portrayal of the parent generation as victimised in order to legitimate what was to come next: economic reform (Rofel, 2007). Yet, the criticism of the CR in this scar literature is not comprehensive (Lee & Dutrait, 2001). While it emphasises how harsh the material and natural conditions were, there is little public criticism or examination of the cultural and social disturbances of that time (Rofel, 2007). This is so even though the Chinese government did engage in introspection and allowed some criticism of actions and agendas during the GLF and the CR (Shambaugh, 2008).

The remembrance of hardship during the GLF and CR time relates to a dominant narrative pattern in modern Chinese history, that of speaking bitterness (*yiku*忆苦). Ge (2016) argued that there is a historical heritage to this pattern, and that it dictates the content of scar literature. A collective narrative of blood and tears is formed by local stories of personal suffering through 'speaking bitterness'. As Ge (2016) claimed, along with appreciating sweetness (*sitian*思甜), yiku embodies the yin–yang dualism of the I Ching (yin symbolises femininity; yang symbolises masculinity). Yin intertwines with yang just as yiku comes together with sitian. Yiku and sitian constitute the official historical practice of feeling grateful for the sweetness of the present by recalling the bitterness of the past (Rofel, 2007). Indeed, this narrative plays a major role in constructing legitimacy for the governmentality of the economic reform initiated in 1978 and rejecting some of the previous policies. By remembering the parents' bitter experiences during GLF and CR, participants are able to rationalise their endeavours to help their parents achieve a complete and satisfying construction of the self in the economic reform era. Parents' sacrifices in the past enable participants' filial care in the present, even though it might mean more difficulties encountered in the endeavour to fulfil filial responsibilities in current Chinese society.

Complexity of Discourse of Filial Piety

Ikels's (2004) claim that filial piety in rural China may not be cultural anymore is an overstatement; for my participants, at least, filial piety was not only practical but also one of the most important ways of (and resources for) constructing their sense of self. Although they might not be as privileged as their urban counterparts or as educated as the younger generation, they could take pride in being filial (Lin, 2013). In assuming their role as caregivers, participants also gained a personal reputation of being filial in their rural communities and among friends and family. Filial piety continued to be a cultural and non-material resource that my participants drew from.

In recent years, traditional filial piety can be seen as negatively influenced by perceived neoliberal 'modernity'. Such modernity depicts modernised personalities as being well educated, metropolitan, well mannered, neoliberal market career-oriented, and so on, while migrant peasant workers are portrayed as being old-fashioned or backward, not progressive, not belonging to the metropolitan city (Kipnis, 2007). This has alienated lower socio-economic social groups, including migrant peasant workers (Jacka, 2009; Zhu, 2001).

The discourse of filial piety enabled participants to make sense of themselves despite their marginalised social position (Lin, 2013). It allowed participants to rationalise their care behaviours and collective filial perceptions (Lin, 2013). As Song (2008) claimed, culture cannot exist without people's deliberate creation, and it serves a certain purpose for people. Filial piety as a cultural norm, to a certain extent, was imagined temporally to accommodate the current needs of participants. This imagining was both an individual and collective societal undertaking. Therefore, subjective filial piety acted like glue for participants. It sustained them against a backdrop of painful memories and experiences of the GLF and CR and enabled them to maintain a somewhat imaginary continuous intergenerational network of relationships.

As discussed in Chapter 4, the relationality of the filial discourse also emerged from and acted to form this network of relationships. Migrant peasant workers drew strength and a sense of power from the relationality of the filial self. Filial piety became foundational for participants' identity construction and the formation of their sense of relationship with their family and society. Several participants expressed similar ideas, such as 'we only exist because of our parents' (P1). Their identity was relational to their parents. The relational self of filial piety was not only animated by the self-interested actions of the participants in terms of educating the next generation and fostering their own reputation. Because filial piety was a moral imperative, its practice was also necessary for participants' self-respect.

Action/Practice-Oriented Discursiveness and Its Importance

There is common ground between Chinese philosophy and Foucauldian discourse theory in this regard. According to Zhang (2015), Foucault took great interest in people's daily life and practices. Foucault strongly stated his preference for investigating regimes of practice, not just theories, institutions, or ideologies (Foucault, 1980). Many ancient Chinese philosophers, including many renowned neo-Confucianists, debated whether practice comes before knowledge or whether knowledge comes before practice. Ultimately, no matter which comes first, these debates provide evidence that Chinese philosophers heavily valued both action and practice. Most ancient Chinese philosophers valued action and practice in social interactions (Feng, 1995; Song, 2008). The tradition of valuing action and practice has inevitably had a huge impact on discourses of filial piety, and continues to be influential, as can be seen in my participants' comments.

Most of my participants did not know how to describe the meaning of being filial towards their parents in fancy language. They did not know how to make direct statements such as 'I love you' to their parents. Their alternative emphasis on 'eating well and dressing well' also indicated their adherence to the tradition of valuing action/practice. In the participants' minds, their understanding of filial piety was embodied in enabling their parents to eat well and dress well. Enabling parents to eat well and dress well required practice and action rather than merely providing comforting words and emotional support. The concept of enabling parents to eat well and dress well emerged from the discursive construction of parental sacrifice. In the parental sacrifice discourse, parents did not eat well or dress well at all during the GLF and CR. By engaging in practices that ensured their parents ate and dressed well now, participants could repay the suffering their parents endured during the GLF and CR. This is not to say that the participants were not concerned with their parents' emotional and other non-material health and happiness; rather, they endeavoured to enable their parents to achieve this well-being through deeds. Some of them, such as P7, said, 'I don't know how to explain—I just know how to do my duties as a son/daughter'. Participants were providing answers and explaining what filial piety was to them by pointing out how they valued the actions and practices that embodied it.

The government-promoted public filial discourse might hinder participants from asking for help. It is rather evident from participants' interviews that they had limited faith in the likelihood of obtaining public support for the care of their parents. Many scholars such as Lan (2002) and Lai (2010) have claimed that filial piety is an obstacle to Chinese people asking for assistance from the government or support agencies. However, asking for help may not necessarily contradict filial morality and performance. As a scholar in human services, I would like to think that to understand and question the filial discursive construction of not asking for help may create conditions in which it becomes possible for people like my participants to carry out actions that make it easier for them to be caregivers. Once discursive constructions are revealed, policymakers and human service practitioners may more readily work towards changes that support filial caregiving without damaging people's filial dignity and pride in taking care of their elders.

As a matter of fact, it was because of the tradition of philosophical emphasis on action/practice in China that Marxism could become and can still remain, at least in the written political agenda, the leading ideology. Chairman Mao once asked where all correct ideas come from, later answering that they come from social practice (Bachman, 2006). According to Fang and Zhao (2004), Chinese society was fertile ground for pragmatically fashioned Marxism to flourish. That is so because both Chinese philosophical tradition and Marxism value action/practice (Cheng, 2013); this common emphasis on action/practice enabled Marxist ideology to thrive in an ancient land for many years.

The Second Research Question: How Are Chinese Migrant Workers Affected by Changes in Discourses of Filial Piety in Current Chinese Society?

The second research question deals with the idea of change. A brief analysis of the genealogy of filial piety in Chinese history (see Chapter 3) reveals that the content of filial piety has been constantly evolving. In the current Chinese context, how does change affect filial perceptions? Foucault's genealogy explores the history of discourse on the topic as a way of understanding the present discourse of filial piety (Foucault, 1978). In this section, I will explain the changes that have occurred in the discourse of filial piety from a Foucauldian point of view.

Chinese Modernity (Chineseness) and Change. When terms such as traditional and cultural filial piety are employed, what do the words tradition and culture actually mean? Tradition and culture reference both the past and the present. Is there already an underlying assumption evident in this wording that tradition has or will be diminished in a progressive western modernised world? In her seminal essay 'Tradition and Patronage in Early India', Thapar (1994) has suggested that tradition is an invention constructed to support contemporary purposes. Exploration of the history of a tradition is 'an attempt... to read the present in terms of the past by writing the past in terms of the present' (Lindstrom, 1982, p. 317). The past is imagined in the service of a present purpose. Tradition is not something created in the past but rather presents unlimited possibilities in the future on which it is drawn (Kleinberg, 2012). According to Cassirer (1972), concepts such as tradition and culture are meaningless unless the philosophies and theories of historical philosophers and thinkers are hermeneutically studied and explained in their relevant contexts. This hermeneutical explanation is endless because we are bound to change our mind (or version of the past) each time our contextualised vision and hence interpretation change (Cassirer, 1972). Thus, modernity is basically the epochalisation of history—dividing time into the traditional past and the modern present plus future.

There are no objective meanings and facts existing in the past because these meanings and facts depend on the present from which they are perceived (Foucault, 1978). In a way, the past has to interact with the present. Past and present are not separate but rather intertwined in a dynamic and complex whole. The forgetting of the GLF and CR is imagined in the present to serve the current filial discourse. Thus, history may turn abruptly through the use of mechanisms of forgetting and imagining. However, this does not necessarily mean that there is no connection between before and after; a highly practised and embedded culture refuses to disappear in a blink of an eye, especially in China with a continuous history over 5,000 years (Jing, 1996; Wang, 2010). Its ever-changing dynamic nature creates multiple realities of a particular cultural discourse (filial piety in this case) during any given period of time.

In some simplistic conceptualisations, the past represents something old, traditional, and cultural while the present presents something new, modern, and liberal. In current Chinese society, the 'past' and 'present' coexist as an interconnected whole, and in this research they come together in the current filial discourse. Some sinological scholars might question why a western methodology has been employed in Chinese research—and I was indeed questioned about that at a sociology conference during my Ph.D. studies (Liang, 2012). In return one might ask why *not* employ a western methodology, since western modernity is already perceived to be prevailing in Chinese society by many contemporary Confucian and Taoist scholars (Wang, 2010).

Chineseness is in fact a kind of Chinese modernity that reinvents the past, using some aspects of western modernity but also reshaping them. There have been a few attempts to redefine modernity since the critique of western hegemonic modernity in the last century. Especially in recent years, according to Gerbaudo (2017), western modernity of the last century has become widely criticised following events such as the 2008 economic crisis, refugee crises, and other social and political challenges. In the west, and increasingly worldwide, there is evidence of an unprecedentedly broad anti-globalisation and pro-localisation movement. Eisenstadt (1999) envisaged a multiple modernity that contains unlimited ways of mixing the traditional and the modern through different variations. Argyrou's (2003) concept of reflexive modernity offered a view of reconstructing western modernity in order to form a more sustainable model advocating unity and equality. Beilharz (2000) presented a vision of modernity that is fluid and watery instead of built on solid ground. Modernity did not cease to exist according to those perspectives but has become open to 'new' ways of looking at contemporary issues. Lee (2006) argued that the above three attempts at redefining modernity demonstrate that modernity remains interconnected with global capital and cannot be isolated from the diversified condition of the contemporary world. The construction of current Chineseness is shaped by the complex dynamics of the interplay of Chinese daily practices, Chinese philosophies, and western modernity.

The influences identified above on the quality of Chineseness, and the complexity of those influences, were evident in the participants' comparisons of the past (mainly the GLF and CR) and the present. Some participants praised the material affluence and infrastructural improvements they experienced or perceived to exist in the present (for example, improved health services for treating diseases such as cancer), compared to the hardship and material deprivation they identified as having existed in the past. By contrast, some participants (such as P3) expressed nostalgia for family co-residency and (his socially constructed perception of) past stronger emotional bonding. All participants expressed a strong will to follow traditional and cultural filial piety imperatives that required them to provide care for their parents in need. However, many of them also commented on the difficulties they encountered in doing so, mainly imposed by modern challenges such as long commuting distances, strict employment conditions for taking leave, and financial issues.

Another example of such complex Chinese and western influences was reflected in many participants' expressed wish to enable their parents to travel to big cities. Travel represented something different and new (Norman, 2013). Most of the participants wanted to take their parents to the big cities, which they perceived to be 'better' and different from the rural hometowns from which they came. Here, my participants yearned for something new in the big cities, something modern, as they said. At the same time, their desire to gift such costly, and in reality usually unattainable, modern travel experiences to their parents before they died also reflected the high value they placed on something old, namely filial piety. To be somewhere new and different perhaps held out the offer of a means by which their parents might say goodbye to the painful memories of the GLF and CR. Moreover, such a gift might help ease the fear and guilt of losing their parents and losing the opportunity to repay the parental 'sacrifice'. Such examples show how contradictory and complex current filial discourse is when it is contextualised through Chinese migrant peasant workers' experiences. Perhaps this is a new form of Chineseness where filial piety could become entangled with consumerism without any apparent contradiction for my participants.

Filial discourse is altered as Chineseness and western modernity continue to reconfigure themselves interactively in current Chinese society. On the one hand, China has morphed into a market-oriented modern society, one whose agricultural society, claimed to be the foundational context for traditional filial piety, is no more (Cheung & Kwan, 2009; Ikels, 2004; Miao, 2015; Poškaitė, 2014). On the other hand, my participants still embraced filial piety as if it had not changed; indeed, many of them said filial piety was similar now to how it was practised in the past. In the process of internalising an 'unchanged' filial piety there is a need for imagination, especially to support the idea of a continuity of filial piety during the GLF and CR. And there is a need to internalise this imagination of a filial past that is continuous with the present because in China there is no equivalent to the western welfare state to provide for eldercare and social security, and because adult children need to retain a strong reciprocal relationship with their parents for practical reasons, including to care for their children when they go to work. The political and public discourse also needs this imagination to be embedded in the population to avoid the huge and possibly unsupportable financial costs of caring for a growing older population. There is a need for such imaginations of a filial past as western modernity gradually loses its charm and domination in Chinese society and as China increasingly becomes more economically powerful in the world (Buzan, 2010).

Is Parental Sacrifice Something New? As mentioned in Chapter 8, most participants explained that they felt there would be a change in filial practice in the next generation. They predicted that the younger generation would not be as filial as they were because younger people did not understand what hardship means. For example, P7 explained that his mother had limited living resources in the years of the GLF and CR and their aftermath. Compared to the resources that his generation had access to due to the success of the economic reforms, his mother's generation experienced much less material comfort. This comparison contributed to the idea or perception of sacrifice. Even though P7's generation had not endured as much hardship as his parents' generation, his generation started to invest more in their children's generation (e.g., financially). Perhaps the increased investment will form into a perception of sacrifice for the next generation, or at least in the near future. This raises a question of whether parental sacrifice is a newly invented discourse or a more deeply embedded and enduring one that ensures filial piety remains a prevalent cultural force. It is possible that the perception and discourse of sacrifice have been long present historically and will continue to be there in the future.

According to Manning and Wemheuer (2011, p. 2), China has been 'a land of famine'. They mention numerous famines occurring from the late Qing dynasty close to the end of the nineteenth century through to the formation of the Republic of China in the early twentieth century, the Japanese invasion period in the 1930s and 1940s, and the GLF famine. Millions of people died of hunger in those famines. Hardship caused by extreme lack of material resources is not a phenomenon limited to the GLF and CR era (Manning & Wemheuer, 2011; Song et al., 2009).

Most participants appreciated what economic reform had brought them, namely the opportunity to 'eat well' and 'dress well'. Most participants described their filial responsibilities as involving enabling parents to eat well and dress well (which, for some participants, involved sending money to them when they needed it), in almost those exact words. I was not surprised by my participants' stories. I myself had been educated with numerous similar tales of hardship by my mother and other family elders when I was a child. My mother told me there was barely any food or clothing for her when she was a child (at the end of the CR). Her father died a few years after the start of economic reforms in 1978 and she expressed her regret that her father never was able to experience the better life that she is experiencing now. It was not until later, however, when I began to analyse the stories that my participants (and my mother) told, that I realised their discursive functions.

Scar literature and the tradition of *yiku sitian* indicate that 'speaking bitterness' may not be something new. Ancient stories, such as that of *mengmu sanqian* 孟母三迁 from over 2,000 years ago relating how Mencius's mother moved three times to better her son's education (Li, 2008), indicate that the perception of the value of parental sacrifice already existed in ancient times. It is not invented during or after Cultural Revolution. These discursive traditions are likely to derive from cultural and moral values that existed many years ago (Rofel, 2007). In another example, parental sacrifice discourse also enabled the participants to follow the important Chinese tradition of honouring the dead. There is an old Chinese saying, 'The dead person matters most' (*sizheweida*, 死者为大), which means nobody can compete with a dead person (Xu, 2007). The dead represent the ancestors who gave us life, knowledge, and humanity, and without them, we would not exist (Xu, 2007). To memorialise the suffering of the dead is therefore essential in Chinese cultural perception (Xu, 2007). For the participants, their parents were dying and would soon become venerated figures. From this perspective, we may consider that the perception of sacrifice is not something invented in the current Chinese context but that has existed since ancient times.

Over time, people may experience and express ideas about parental sacrifice differently as contextual factors change. For example, P7 expressed a sentiment that would have been frowned upon only a short time ago. He said, 'No matter how filial we are, it can't compete with two old people caring for each other [and] washing each other's feet and face and such.... I hope he [P7's father] can find someone soon'. Just a decade ago, whether a widow(er) should get remarried was a controversial issue for the children (Huang, 2012). Yet for some children finding a spouse for their widowed parent has now become one of their filial responsibilities, showing that these responsibilities are shaped by different social circumstances. Therefore, the role of sacrifice discourse in maintaining cultural and social integrity may be deeply embedded even if the content of stories might be different from the stories that were told 200 or 2,000 years ago.

A Way Forward for China's Ageing Population and Family Caregiving

How might the suggestion mentioned above—that what is needed is action/practice-focused policy—be taken forward in the current Chinese context? On the basis of this research, a starting point involves raising awareness of two discourses of filial piety: parental sacrifice and forgetting. This requires that the forgotten has to be remembered. The technique of remembering the forgotten is also connected to the Confucian way of cultivation of the self and the Foucauldian concept of parrhesia.

Time to Remember?

Without remembering, the concept of forgetting would cease to exist (Krondorfer, 2008). According to Nora (1989), history is often remembered in modern literature. However, there are often no in-depth historical accounts or references in those memories (Krondorfer, 2008). In order to gather an in-depth account of history, the concept of forgetting needs to be appreciated and promoted to the centre of the study of history and of historiography as much as remembering does (Krondorfer, 2008). If one forgets, one can only know whether one has forgotten or not through remembering. If one cannot remember, at least partial fragments, one will never know that one has forgotten anything. Through constant reflexive thoughts moving between forgetting and remembering, the depths of history are thus reached. Indeed, history is remembered in the present, while many alternative historical accounts are forgotten in the process. In this research, forgetting discourse was the adopted concept to make sense of participants' filial narratives. Remembering could not be separated from forgetting. Forgetting was understood from participants' statements that showed how a participant remembered to forget about the past.

Anecdotes and academic literature about the CR can still be found online. Things that are forgotten have been known at some time and may again be knowable. Recent history may be easily forgotten (Halperin, 1998). Indeed, a recent national tragic period of time might be emotionally difficult to remember on a personal level (Krondorfer, 2008), let alone when other forces that encourage forgetting, such as a public discourse of forgetting. Perhaps it is time to start to remember that which has been forgotten. My mother started to remember and pass on her knowledge and stories to me. Even though she did this mainly for the sake of my PhD education, this proved that she could still retrieve the forgotten. This suggests these stories are waiting to be told. The concept of remembering to forget is not newly invented in this research. According to Schaumann (2008), grandchildren of Nazi victims and perpetrators appeared to connect with what had been forgotten immediately after the Second World War when their parents, who were the children of that era, found it difficult to remember and easier to forget.

Discussions with P4 and P15 about 'those years' in Chapter 8 suggested a possibility of remembering a past. In these participants' accounts, filial practices during the GLF and CR were at the very least not perfect. While they did not mention stories about parents being disobeyed and confronted by children, their accounts were nonetheless ambivalent, suggesting that they might become able to access more unsettling versions of history in the future. Foucault, in his book *Nietzsche, Genealogy, History*, valued the occurrence of chance in human lives (Foucault, 1978). This chance he was talking about makes future changes possible. In this case, a recognition of imperfect filial perception or practices during the GLF and CR could elicit a remembering of the forgotten.

According to Rumsfeld (2002, p.1),

> There are known knowns. These are things we know that we know. There are known unknowns. That is to say, there are things that we now know we don't know. But there are also unknown unknowns. These are things we do not know we don't know.

Even though it might be difficult, people are starting to remember the 'known unknowns'. In addition to P4 and P15, several other participants also talked about 'those years', as mentioned in the two previous chapters.

The notion of the relational self of filial piety that was discussed in Chapter 4, draws attention to the complexity of relationships between the individual and others. The complexity of coexisting neoliberal and non-neoliberal features in the China of today also demonstrates the complexity of contextual influences on changing filial practices. Social transformation in China is far more complex than can be simply explained by reference to neoliberalism or to the political agenda of the 'modernisation project'. According to Rofel (2007), Chinese people are strongly motivated to be autonomous, entrepreneurial, and global, but this does not mean they are not simultaneously traditional and familial. This research showed how the current understanding of the discourse of filial piety is pivotally shaped by the forgetting of recent history.

One has to remember in order to realise that one has forgotten something (Epstein, 2001). The concept of forgetting differs from selectively choosing to ignore. As shown in the words of Rumsfeld (2002) at the beginning of this section, if one does not know that one does not know, there will be no remembrance or forgetting at all. If one knows one has forgotten something, this means there is a possibility that the forgotten can be recalled at some stage. Forgetting affects how one imagines one's past experiences or perceptions (Gordon, 2014). It is remembering that reimagines the past. Remembering is not of the exact past but a forgotten and then reconstituted past. In this research, participants were starting to be able to remember the forgotten. One participant (P3) said she thought the next generation was more filial, countering widely held beliefs. This participant might start to remember that filial piety was heavily criticised during the GLF and CR.

For my participants, parental sacrifice and forgetting discourses were constructed as mechanisms that mainly functioned to strengthen filial perception and practice in the complex Chinese context of the present time. However, as also mentioned in Chapter 8, forgetting was identified to occur in different generations, and many of my participants worried that the younger generation would not be as filial because they do not understand what *xinku* (辛苦, hardship) is. The parents of the younger generation (born after the late 1980s and 1990s) would not have experienced the GLF and CR. Therefore, the discursive construction of parental sacrifice and forgetting would lose some ground. In order to maintain filial practices and perceptions, it is perhaps time to start to remember the forgotten aspects of events that occurred during 'those years'. Remembering that this recent history was a discursive construction by both the Chinese government and Chinese people, such remembering would consequently enable a different set of content to emerge on the basis of which a new construction of filial piety could be built. As discussed earlier, while discursive construction might still be the same, the content will change.

We often simplify in order to understand (Tsoukas, 2017). Otherwise, the interlinked connectedness of social conditions and the relational self that is situated within those can hardly be articulated and grasped. Just as this book simplifies filial discourse, participants simplified their life stories when they spoke. Did stories and meanings become lost in this simplification? The process of simplification also involves forgetting. Forgetting facilitates simplification. Perhaps, forgetting discourse does not only exist in the current Chinese filial discourse but is an important aspect of more general social phenomena and discourses. Remembering the forgotten provides a way to reduce the oversimplification of the complexity of filial discourse in today's Chinese society when it becomes necessary to sharpen our focus and draw attention to certain aspects of a social problem that requires creative solutions. The unsettling interplay of Chineseness and westernisation has to be understood first and then dealt with. Filial piety is not just an issue concerning population ageing and eldercare; it relates to a broader unsettling of Chineseness in a transitioning modern society. In the next section, the implications of the study findings for filial piety and its extended suggestions on Chineseness will be discussed.

Cultivation of the Self (Parrhesia)

> *Parrhesia* is a kind of verbal activity where the speaker has a specific relation to truth through frankness, a certain relationship to his own life through danger, a certain relation to himself or other people through criticism … and a specific relation to moral law through freedom and duty.

> More precisely, parrhesia is a verbal activity in which a speaker expresses his personal relationship to truth, and risks his life because he recognizes truth-telling as a duty to improve or help other people (as well as himself). In *parrhesia*, the speaker uses his freedom and chooses frankness instead of persuasion, truth instead of falsehood or silence, the risk of death instead of life and security, criticism instead of flattery, and moral duty instead of self-interest and moral apathy. (Foucault, 1999, p. 5)

According to Besley and Peters (2007), parrhesia is a notion that Foucault borrowed from ancient Greek and Roman times. Parrhesia's several traits are identified in Foucault's summary of the concept above. Firstly, it involves a relationship between the speaker (the parrhesiast), 'the frankly spoken truth, and the listener' (Foucault & Pearson, 2001, p. 23). Secondly, parrhesia presupposes that the parrhesiast speaks a truth that he believes. Thirdly, parrhesia comes with a moral courage that enables parrhesiasts to speak out despite the risk of dangerous consequences. Fourthly, parrhesia functions more as a form of criticism of the other than an explanation of the truth, as the parrhesiasts are always in a less powerful position than the interlocutors. Lastly, parrhesia itself is a duty of telling the truth (Foucault & Pearson, 2001).

According to Mou (2005), Confucianism has had a philosophical focus on cultivation of the self, which appears to be in common with Foucault's notion of parrhesia. Heubel (2008) claimed that the common ground for cultivation of the self between Confucianism and Foucault might enlighten a new way of looking at modernity. For Heubel (2008), there is no point in deconstructing western modernity as it has become a global phenomenon in various unique ways in different cultures. A new methodology is needed to understand what modern Chineseness is, for example. According to Heubel (2008), a new methodology can possibly be located in the common ground between Foucault's parrhesia and the Confucian cultivation of the self, and the use of Chinese language for the translation of western philosophies and social theories. According to Wang (2008) and Wang (2016), in the Confucian conceptualisation of the cultivation of the self, *junzi*—the ideal type of human being—also has a duty to tell the truth and has no fear of criticising the person in power regardless of his safety. Chen (2017) distinguished a fundamental difference between Foucault and the Confucian concept of cultivation of the self: in Confucianism, the cultivation of the self is at the heart of politics and thereby encouraged, whereas Foucault mainly saw parrhesia as a technique for *care of the self* and resisting politics. Both Chen (2017) and Heubel (2008) identified that the commonly overwhelming interest in cultivation of the self shines a light not only on matters of Chinese modernity (e.g., how to define Chineseness in contemporary society) but also on specific social issues.

Parrhesia links closely with my research in four respects. Firstly, as discussed in the last section, parrhesia provides a way of remembering what happened in the past (during the GLF and the CR). The discourse of forgetting can be reconstructed through parrhesia by remembering (telling) the 'truth' (the which was forgotten).

Secondly, parrhesia also challenges the public forgetting discourse in terms of its lack of practical supporting policies and the government's forgetting of traumatic events that occurred in those years. The Chinese government did engage in a process of self-criticism after the CR (Kleinman & Kleinman, 1994) and has made efforts to improve its welfare system in recent years (Ringen & Ngok, 2017). It is perhaps time to enable parrhesia in its own political discourse so that more unbiased criticism may take place and enhance understanding of the government's past and practical policies may be enabled.

Thirdly, in Foucault's care of the self, parrhesia was a technique for achieving freedom from discursive constraints. In China, not telling parents about their cancer diagnosis is common practice. This practice is problematic for both parents and children. For example, children may not be able to gain emotional closure by saying a proper goodbye to their parents or receive emotional support and comfort from talking to their parents and other family and friends. Parents are powerless in the decision-making process concerning their own health and death. Their right to provide informed consent and receive information are disrespected within this practice of secrecy. Applying the practice of parrhesia does not determine that children should definitely and imminently tell their parents about their impending death, but perhaps involves a negotiation between generations.

Finally, parrhesia is a function of researchers, theorists, and academics, including social scientists who study human services; their role is to bring to light hidden perspectives and not shirk in delivering what may at times be uncomfortable messages in order to create opportunities for change.

Conclusion

In this chapter, the discussion opened with a focus on the two research questions. The first research question investigated the mechanism participants employed to interact with (negotiate and employ) current filial discourses in their journeys of caring for their parents with terminal cancer. The identified parental sacrifice and forgetting discourses contributed greatly in terms of understanding how migrant peasant workers made sense of their caring experiences for parents with terminal cancer under the umbrella of filial discourse. Indeed, the mechanisms afforded by parental sacrifice and forgetting discourses were required to enable the participants to negotiate their caring roles in the face of contextual changes in current Chinese society.

Chinese philosophical discourse of filial piety has a major investment in action and practice. Such interests were evident in my participants' comments and stories. An action/practice orientation is also in line with the spirit of the discipline of human services. Such an orientation sheds light on the need to address future policy implications in order to facilitate filial care. An action-oriented filial discourse is meaningful in current Chinese society, where it is becoming better recognised that western European welfare states do not provide appropriate models to emulate.

The second major question posed in my research related to the changes that might have occurred in my participants' perception of filial practice. Neoliberalisation and modernisation have been blamed for changes in filial practices since the start of economic reform in 1978 in China. Both neoliberalisation and modernisation appeared to reflect an overweening alignment with western modernity. However, there is an undeniably persistent Chinese tradition and culture that remains evident in Chinese society. Parental sacrifice and forgetting discourses revealed the complexity of current Chineseness. A sense of change in Chinese society was discussed in this chapter in relation to the notion of Chineseness, which presents a new form of Chinese modernity that draws some ideas from and is influenced by western modernity. How changes in the discourse of filial piety affected the participants was the focus of the discussion relating to the second research question. Changes in the current Chinese context were reflected in fears that the next generation of Chinese would be less filial.

Chinese society today carries a somewhat confused sense of 'traditional' filial piety. Both the participants and I as a researcher had difficulties when attempting to make sense of changes in filial perceptions and practices. The ancient Chinese philosophies may provide a way to incorporate techniques for care of the self and the construction of free ethical subjects that parallel the way Foucault drew on the strength of parrhesia from ancient Greek and Roman genealogical literature.

References

Anagnost, A. (2004). The corporeal politics of quality (*suzhi*). *Public Culture, 16*(2), 189–208. https://doi.org/10.1215/08992363-16-2-189

Andersen, N. A. (2003). *Discursive analytical strategies: Understanding Foucault, Koselleck, Laclau, Luhmann*. Policy Press.

Argyrou, V. (2003). 'Reflexive modernization' and other mythical realities. *Anthropological Theory, 3*(1), 27–41. https://doi.org/10.1177/1463499603003001750

Bachman, D. (2006). *Bureaucracy, economy, and leadership in China: The institutional origins of the Great Leap Forward*. Cambridge University Press.

Beilharz, P. (2000). *Zygmunt Bauman: Dialectic of modernity*. Sage.

Besley, T., & Peters, M. (2007). *Subjectivity & truth: Foucault, education, and the culture of self*. Peter Lang.

Buzan, B. (2010). China in international society: Is 'peaceful rise' possible? *The Chinese Journal of International Politics, 3*(1), 5–36. https://doi.org/10.18359/ries.1869

Cassirer, E. (1972). *An essay on man: An introduction to a philosophy of human culture* (Vol. 52). Yale University Press.

Chen, X. (2017). Cultivation of self: The possibility of communication between Foucault and Chinese philosophy 皆以修身为本——福柯与中国修身哲学沟通的可能性. *Hubei Social Science 湖北社会科学* (7), 104–110. http://fbsf.Chinajournal.net.cn

Cheng, M. (2013). Mao's Marxist revolution on a Chinese cultural foundation 论毛泽东创新马克思主义的中国文化基础. *Bejing University Publisher (Social Science) 北京大学学报(哲学社会科学版), 50*(6), 5–13. http://bjdxxb.xueshu.com/

Cheung, C. K., & Kwan, A.Y.-H. (2009). The erosion of filial piety by modernisation in Chinese cities. *Ageing & Society, 29*(2), 179–198. https://doi.org/10.1017/S0144686X08007836

Eisenstadt, S. N. (1999). *Fundamentalism, sectarianism, and revolution: The Jacobin dimension of modernity*. Cambridge University Press.

Epstein, J. (2001). Remember to forget: The problem of traumatic cultural memory. In J. Epstein & L. H. Lefkovitz (Eds.), *Shaping losses: Cultural memory and the Holocaust* (pp. 186–204). University of Illinois Press. http://ifdpublishing.com/blog/?page_id=2057

Fang, H., & Zhao, Z. (2004). Marxism and the Chinese cultural spirit: Cultural interpretation of Chineseness of Marxism 马克思主义与中国文化精神--马克思主义中国化的文化解释. *Northwest Normal University Publishing (Social Science) 西北师范大学学报(社会科学版), 41*(2), 55–58. http://xbbjb.nwnu.edu.cn

Feng, Y. (1995). *History of Chinese philosophy 中国哲学史*. Zhonghua Shuju.

Forkel, I., & Silbereisen, R. K. (2001). Family economic hardship and depressed mood among young adolescents from former East and West Germany. *American Behavioral Scientist, 44*(11), 1955–1971. https://doi.org/10.1177/00027640121958131

Foucault, M. (1970). *The archaeology of knowledge*. Tavistock.

Foucault, M. (1978). Nietzsche, genealogy, history. *Semiotexte, 3*(1), 78–94.

Foucault, M. (1980). *Language, counter-memory, practice: Selected essays and interviews*. Blackwell.

Foucault, M. (1991). *The Foucault effect: Studies in governmentality*. University of Chicago Press.

Foucault, M. (1999). *Discourse and truth: The problematization of parrhesia; Six lectures given by Michel Foucault at the University of California at Berkeley, October–November 1983*. Retrieved from https://foucault.info/parrhesia/

Foucault, M. (2000). The subject and power. In J. D. Faubion (Ed.), *Power*. The New Press.

Foucault, M., & Pearson, J. (2001). *Fearless speech*. Semiotexte.

Galik, M. (1982). Some remarks on 'literature of the scars' in the People's Republic of China (1977–1979). *Asian and African Studies, 18*, 53–74. http://journals.sagepub.com/home/jas

Ge, X. (2016). A tale of "*ku*" (bitter) v.s. "*tian*" (sweet): Understanding China's "*yiku sitian*" movement in the 1960s and 1970s from the perspective of cultural discourse analysis. Doctoral dissertation, University of Massachusetts.

Gerbaudo, P. (2017). *The mask and the flag: Populism, citizenism and global protest*. Oxford University Press.

Gordon, M. (2014). Between remembering and forgetting. *Studies in Philosophy and Education, 34*(5), 489–295. https://doi.org/10.1007/s11217-014-9451-2

Greenhalgh, S., & Winckler, E. A. (2005). *Governing China's population: From Leninist to neoliberal biopolitics*. Stanford University Press.

Hairong, Y. (2003). Neoliberal governmentality and neohumanism: Organizing suzhi/value flow through labor recruitment networks. *Cultural Anthropology, 18*(4), 493–523. https://doi.org/10.1525/can.2003.18.4.493

Halperin, D. M. (1998). Forgetting Foucault: Acts, identities, and the history of sexuality. *Representations, 63*, 93–120. https://doi.org/10.2307/2902919

Heubel, F. (2008). Cross-cultural critique and contemporary Chinese language philosophy: A reflection on the methodology of researching the late Michel Foucault 跨文化批判与当代汉语哲学——晚期福柯研究的方法论反思. *Scholarly Research* 学术研究 (3), 5–13. http://mall.cnki.net/magazine/magalist/XSYJ.htm

Huang, Y. (2012). Remarriage, gender, and life course in contemporary inland rural China. *Journal of Comparative Family Studies, 43*(2), 313–330. https://doi.org/10.3138/jcfs.43.2.313

Ikels, C. (2004). *Filial piety: Practice and discourse in contemporary East Asia*. Stanford University Press.

Jacka, T. (2009). Cultivating citizens: *Suzhi* (quality) discourse in the PRC. *Positions: Asia Critique, 17*(3), 523–536. https://doi.org/10.1215/10679847

Jing, J. (1996). *The temple of memories: History, power, and morality in a Chinese village*. Stanford University Press.

Kipnis, A. (2007). Neoliberalism reified: Suzhi discourse and tropes of neoliberalism in the People's Republic of China. *Journal of the Royal Anthropological Institute, 13*(2), 383–400. https://doi.org/10.1111/j.1467-9655.2007.00432.x

Kleinberg, E. (2012). Back to where we've never been: Heidegger, Levinas, and Derrida on tradition and history. *History and Theory, 51*(4), 114–135. https://doi.org/10.1111/j.1468-2303.2012.00650.x

Kleinman, A., & Kleinman, J. (1994). How bodies remember: Social memory and bodily experience of criticism, resistance, and delegitimation following China's Cultural Revolution. *New Literary History, 25*(3), 707–723. https://doi.org/10.2307/469474

Krondorfer, B. (2008). Is forgetting reprehensible? Holocaust remembrance and the task of oblivion. *The Journal of Religious Ethics, 36*(2), 233–267. https://doi.org/10.1111/j.1467-9795.2008.00345.x

Lai, D. W. (2010). Filial piety, caregiving appraisal, and caregiving burden. *Research on Aging, 32*(2), 200–223. https://doi.org/10.1177/0164027509351475

Lan, P. C. (2002). Subcontracting filial piety: Elder care in ethnic Chinese immigrant families in California. *Journal of Family Issues, 23*(7), 812–835. https://doi.org/10.1177/019251302236596

Lee, G., & Dutrait, N. (2001). Conversations with Gao Xingjian: The first "Chinese" winner of the Nobel Prize for Literature. *The China Quarterly, 167*(167), 738–748. https://doi.org/10.1017/S0009443901000419

Lee, R. L. M. (2006). Reinventing modernity: Reflexive modernization vs liquid modernity vs multiple modernities. *European Journal of Social Theory, 9*(3), 355–368. https://doi.org/10.1177/1368431006065717

Li, L. (2008). The contemporary value of the education principle of Mencius's mother孟母家教原则及其当代价值研究. *Education Exploration 教育探索, 10*, 006.

Liang, D. (2012). *School of Guoxue: The origins of Chinese studies 国学堂:国学溯源*. Science Publisher 科学出版社.

Lin, X. (2013). *Gender, modernity and male migrant workers in China: Becoming a 'modern' man*. Routledge.

Lindstrom, L. (1982). Leftamap Kastom: The political history of tradition on Tanna Vanuatu. *The Australian Journal of Anthropology, 13*(4), 316–329. https://doi.org/10.1111/j.1835-9310.1982.tb00997.x

Ma, L. (2009). China's authoritarian capitalism: Growth, elitism and legitimacy. *International Development Planning Review, 31*(1), i–xii. https://doi.org/10.3828/idpr.31.1.1

Manning, K. E., & Wemheuer, F. (2011). *Eating bitterness: New perspectives on China's Great Leap Forward and famine*. UBC Press.

Miao, C. (2015). The evolution of filial piety in ancient China and its influence on neighboring countries: Taking the classic of filial piety as the chief source. *Asian Social Science, 11*(12), 319–325. https://doi.org/10.5539/ass.v11n12p319

Mou, J., Griffiths, S. M., Fong, H., & Dawes, M. G. (2013). Health of China's rural–urban migrants and their families: A review of literature from 2000 to 2012. *British Medical Bulletin, 106*(1), 19–43. https://doi.org/10.1093/bmb/ldt016

Mou, Z. (2005). *Life's knowledge 生命的学问*. SanMing ShuJu 三民书局.

Nora, P. (1989). Between memory and history: *Les lieux de mémoire*. *Representations, 26*, 7–24. https://doi.org/10.2307/2928520

Norman, A. (2013). *Journeys and destinations: Studies in travel, identity, and meaning*. Cambridge Scholars.

Poškaitė, L. (2014). Filial piety (*xiao* 孝) for the contemporary and global world. *Asian Studies, 2*(1), 99–114. https://doi.org/10.4312/as.2014.2.1.99-114

Ringen, S., & Ngok, K. (2017). What kind of welfare state is emerging in China? In I. Yi (Ed.), *Towards universal health care in emerging economies* (pp. 213–237). Springer.

Rofel, L. (2007). *Desiring China: Experiments in neoliberalism, sexuality, and public culture*. Duke University Press.

Rumsfeld, D. (2002, February 12). *US Department of Defense news briefing*. Retrieved from http://archive.defense.gov

Schaumann, C. (2008). *Memory matters: Generational responses to Germany's Nazi past in recent women's literature* (Vol. 4). Walter de Gruyter.

Shambaugh, D. L. (2008). *China's communist party: Atrophy and adaptation*. University of California Press.

Song, S., Wang, W., & Hu, P. (2009). Famine, death, and madness: Schizophrenia in early adulthood after prenatal exposure to the Chinese Great Leap Forward famine. *Social Science & Medicine, 68*(7), 1315–1321. https://doi.org/10.1016/j.socscimed.2009.01.027

Song, Z. (2008). *Chinese traditional philosophical discussion 中国传统哲学通*. People's University of China Press.

Thapar, R. (1994). *Cultural transaction and early India: Tradition and patronage*. Oxford University Press.

Tsoukas, H. (2017). Don't simplify, complexify: From disjunctive to conjunctive theorizing in organization and management studies. *Journal of Management Studies, 54*(2), 132–153. https://doi.org/10.1111/joms.12219

Wang, D. (2010). *The fall of humanity 人类的没落* . Xianxi People's Publisher.

Wang, D. (2016). The one with no fear has a heart of fear: Three fears of Junzi and its educational purpose for youth 无畏者怀有的敬畏之心——君子三畏及对青年的借鉴意义. *Social Science 社会科学:全文版* (12), 00047. http://www.cqvip.com/QK/72177X/

Wang, L. (2008). The Confucian concept of Junzi and the thought of Zhongyong 孔子的君子观与中庸思想. *Hubei Second Normal College Publisher 湖北第二师范学院学报, 25*(1), 79–80. http://www.eshukan.com

Wang, Y. (2014). *Chinese traditional filial piety and contemporary rural family elder care research 中国传统孝道思想与当代农村家庭养老研究*. Qinghai Normal University 青海师范大学.

Wong, N. (1988). *The great chaos: The ten year history of the Cultural Revolution 大动乱的年代:文化大革命十年史* (Vol. 3). People's Publisher of Henan.

Wu, F. (2010). How neoliberal is China's reform? The origins of change during transition. *Eurasian Geography and Economics, 51*(5), 619–631. https://doi.org/10.2747/1539-7216.51.5.619

Xiao, Q. (2001). *Filial piety and Chinese culture*. People's Publications.

Xu, F. (2007). The traumatic memory of anti-rightism 50 years later 五十年后的"反右"创伤记忆. *Contemporary Chinese Research,* 3(98), 20–30. http://www.iccs.cn/

Yan, J. (1999). Evaluation of the argument between "4th May", "Cultural Revolution" and the traditional culture 评"五四","文革"与传统文化的论争. *Chinese and Foreign Culture and Discussion 中外文化与文论, 1*(2), 2–13. http://www.gwyoo.com/qikan/zhengfawenshi/wenhua/201003/354695.html

Zhang, X. (2015). An essay on Foucault's shift towards ethics in his late stage 论福柯晚期思想的伦理转向. *World Philosophy 世界哲学, 3*, 011. http://www.sjzxzz.cn/

Zhu, L. (2001). Collective discrimination and bias: The conflicting interaction between migrant peasant workers and urban residents 群体性偏见与歧视--农民工与市民的磨擦性互动. *Jianghai Academic Periodical 江海学刊* (6), 48–53. http://www.jhxk.cn/CN/volumn/home.shtml

CHAPTER 10

Conclusion

Introduction

From the preceding discussion, it is evident that blaming neoliberal marketisation for changes in filial practices, including a diminished adherence to filial practices in some aspects and in some contexts, is not only overly simplistic but also naïve. Although the Chinese sociopolitical context is not specifically defined in my research, it is obvious that the Chinese political system exhibits an element of non-neoliberalism. Claims that diminishing filial piety is a result of neoliberalisation also overlook the discursive formation of filial piety, and fail to unravel the complexities of its archaeological contextual and historical moulding. In the practical arena, an overgeneralised assumption might induce a political response such as the 'parent-visiting law', which was argued to be, to some extent, ineffective and unworkable by participants in my research. My participants considered this law to be prompted by good intentions to combat a decline in filial piety, but they thought the law to be too general and impractical.

In this final chapter I consider how a thorough examination of the discourse of filial piety can contribute to more suitable suggestions for policymakers. This is important in the Chinese context where informal caregiving remains the main care resource for rural elders. My research examined migrant peasant workers' care experiences for elderly parents suffering from cancer, in relation to their perception of filial piety. I

L. He, *Care Work, Migrant Peasant Families and Discourse of Filial Piety in China*, https://doi.org/10.1007/978-981-16-1880-2_10

undertook this research using a methodology grounded in a Foucauldian discourse analysis (FDA) perspective that was consistent with principles from Chinese philosophy.

This chapter includes three main sections. The first section presents a review of research questions and the main findings. Next follows a section explaining why my research is important. In the final section, I draw on my findings to make recommendations for future research and policies, so as to improve migrant peasant workers' care conditions and better support their filial care practices.

Research Questions and Findings

In this section, I look back at my research aims and objectives and revisit research findings that emerged in my endeavour to answer these two questions below (see also Chapter 9). From the analysis of my collected data, I found that discourses of filial piety shaped and reflected how my participants made sense of care responsibilities and burdens. This reflexive meaning-making process showed how complex the discursive construction of filial piety is. Identification of two important discourses of filial piety—those of parental sacrifice and of forgetting—revealed the process of the discursive construction of filial piety. This construction not only was complex but also revealed itself to be of a pragmatic nature. The discursive construction of filial piety through parental sacrifice and forgetting helps reaffirm filial perceptions and practices in a changing social context since economic reform up to the present. However, among my participants, a deep worry still lingered that filial piety might fall off in a future generation.

Research Questions

My research originally set out to explore the experiences of adult children who care for terminally ill parents living in rural China. Within a short time of commencing the research, it became clear that this caregiving context was interwoven with considerations and practices of filial piety. My research was thus reconceptualised as a study to examine the complex construction of filial piety, in the context of end-of-life care experiences of migrant peasant workers in China who look after parents with terminal cancer. To be more precise, it aimed to explore the following research questions:

How do Chinese migrant workers make sense of caring experiences for parents with terminal cancer? How does their sense-making relate to and reflect discourses of filial piety?
To what extent and how are Chinese migrant workers affected by changes in discourses of filial piety in current Chinese society?

My research objective was to discover what participants' discursive constructions, policy and other documents, and academic literature might reveal about current discourses of filial piety; how these constructions could be understood; how complex discourses of filiality are constructed through various contextual factors; how power relations are mediated between and among governmental discourses and subjective discourses of filial piety, especially when different political agendas contradict each other; and how change is perceived and might be reconciled.

In order to answer these questions, 24 migrant peasant workers were interviewed in a city hospital in Langzhong city. Each open-ended interview lasted one–two hours. At the end of the interview, participants also completed a survey questionnaire, mainly for the purpose of collecting demographic information. This data has been integrated into the findings, for example where participants are described as male or female, and where findings about the economic hardships suffered by participants are discussed. The interviews were audiorecorded, transcribed by both me and a hired professional transcriber, and then translated from Mandarin into English by me. Translations were checked by one of my supervisors who is a native Chinese speaker. Additionally, field notes were made and selected government documents were consulted to deepen the mainly FDA approach, which was complemented by a consideration of gender prompted by readings in critical discourse analysis and underpinned by Chinese philosophical understandings.

Care Responsibilities and Burden in Relation to the Discourses of Filial Piety

The original rationale for this research emerged from a concern for the impacts that end-of-life care experiences have on informal caregivers in China. The palliative and end-of-life care movements have shone a light on the importance of informal caregivers (Li et al., 2011). The contextual factors that are associated with informal caregiving patterns and caregivers' burdens involve many domains of Chinese life and society, such as the relatively inadequate welfare system that provides severely limited pensions and health benefits; insufficient affordable hospital services and lack of resources including lack of home- or community-based support, or even hospital nursing care; lack of dedicated end-of-life care facilities; the one-child policy resulting in a shortage of informal caregivers; and other cultural, socio-economic, and policy factors, including urbanisation resulting in substantial distance between adult children and ill parents (Cohen et al., 2015; Gruijters, 2017a, 2017b; Yang, 2009; Zhang, 2016; Zhu, 2001).

At least some of these contextual factors have more profound influences on rural families than on urban ones. According to Ikels (2004), in rural China, filial piety might not be primarily seen by outsiders as a 'cultural' discourse but might rather be a practical necessity. She found that filial support from children involved a practical exchange of resources with parents who were reciprocally involved in caregiving, such as the rearing of grandchildren (Ikels, 2004). Rural older persons rely on their adult children for financial support due to a lack of social welfare provisions and to their financially disadvantaged position in the market economy (Zhou, 2011). Elders become a 'burden' for their children. According to Zhu (2019), some rural older persons even try to kill themselves when they are diagnosed with terminal illness because they fear that medical expenses could bankrupt their adult children. Some of my participants had to vigorously persuade their parents to accept treatment and stop engaging in strenuous farming duties, measures that were resisted by parents because they wanted to be seen as useful and not burdensome.

As discussed in previous chapters, the changing contextual factors mentioned above interact with the discourse of filial piety in terms of care impacts, sense of care responsibilities, and care burdens. There were several forms of impacts identified from participants' interviews. Emotional impacts and related physical impacts were explained first, in Chapter 6. Participants expressed their sorrow about their parent's illness and imminent death. Some participants felt they were losing someone they had depended on physically, mentally, and emotionally. Such emotional impacts were often associated with physical effects such as sleep deprivation. Other physical impacts, such as physical discomfort and the worsening of one's own health condition, often due to extensive disruption of everyday life routines, were also identified. Financial impact was seen as the biggest 'burden' and financial support was the type of support most desired by many participants. Work-related factors were implicated in the financial strain suffered by migrant workers, including low relative wages paid to rural migrants relative to wages paid to workers whose families originated in the urban areas, long travelling times required for visits due to distance between workplaces and hometowns, excessive work hours, and difficulties in obtaining any form of leave—even unpaid leave—and inequitable policies for leave applications. Additionally, many participants spoke of a sense of unfinished care; unfulfilled wishes, such as to enable parents to travel, especially to big cities, frequently emerged in participants' interviews. This sense of incompleteness connotes difficult-to-process emotions such as regret, guilt, and shame.

The impacts mentioned above might be considered to be responsibilities, burdens, or both. At first in almost all my participants' interviews, participants did not appear to think care was a burden for them, and they asserted that their care experiences did not involve significant negative impacts. However, as we approached the end of the interview and in the subsequent questionnaire stage, where they also had an opportunity to express themselves, many of them began to mention the word 'burden' and speak out about the types of burdens they had to shoulder. The analysis showed that these seemingly paradoxical narratives revealed the discursive formation of filial piety. Early in the interviews, participants appeared to fear that talking about burden might make them look unfilial in my eyes, which would lead to loss of face. As many participants said, it was their 'natural' responsibility to care for their parents. The discourse of *tianjingdiyi* (natural), as discussed in Chapter 7, was identified from participants' explanations of their sense of responsibility. As the interview proceeded to delve into different forms of impacts, they opened up and told me they were experiencing many burdens. However, this discourse did again also appear to be presented, at least in part, in such a way as to show me how filial they were, since despite all of the burdens they faced, they still fulfilled or attempted to fulfil their filial responsibilities.

Discourses of Parental Sacrifice and Forgetting

Intergenerational care for parents from children does not equate to filial piety, but it is an important aspect of filial piety. As discussed in Chapter 3, filial piety and care are often conflated. According to Cheung and Kwan (2009), consequences of urbanisation and a move to a market economy have resulted in negative impacts on care behaviours from adult children towards parents in rural China. Therefore, claims about a decline in filial piety are often based on the changing pattern of family care provided by adult children to parents. Meanwhile, empirical research has also examined the role that filial piety plays in the motivation for family caregiving, and the role that being able to fulfil filial piety responsibilities plays as a factor in the well-being of caregivers (Chan et al., 2012). In my research, discourses of filial piety were intertwined with participants' care for their parents, as demonstrated in the previous section.

For my participants, their caregiving, their contribution to their parents, their respect, and so on, were all aspects of fulfilling filial piety, amounting to more than just responsibilities and instead seen as *Tianjingdiyi* (natural). Furthermore, for my participants, filial piety was also a resource from which they drew support and comfort, enabling them to face the challenges imposed upon them by the current Chinese modernity.

My research successfully identified two mechanisms via which filial piety was (re)constructed despite contravening contextual changes. As discussed in the above section, my participants highly valued filial piety and considered it natural to provide filial care to their parents in need. From the analysis of my data the discursive mechanisms that helped participants to combat negative contextual changes were those constructed around parental sacrifice and forgetting. From the genealogical analysis, both parental sacrifice discourse and forgetting discourse were heavily associated with a period of time: the Great Leap Forward (GLF; 1958–1962) and the Cultural Revolution (CR; 1966–1976). A parental sacrifice discourse enabled participants to 'remember' a parental past life filled with sacrifice and hardship, endured for the sake of raising them and for the wider welfare of the family. A forgetting discourse enabled participants to 'forget' some things, such as their parents' political pursuits and earlier critique of filial piety in 'those' periods in order to enable the current discursive formation of filial piety. The forgetting discourse also incorporates a form of political and public forgetting. The government 'forgets' that it once highly criticised filial piety and tried to erase it from Chinese society. As discussed in Chapter 9, my genealogical analysis and resultant findings drew attention to the impact of the GLF and the CR on the construction of filial care.

Pragmatic Element of Discourse of Filial Piety

A pragmatic element of participants' filial care was detected from the discourse analysis. The discourse of eating and dressing well (discussed in Chapter 7) depicts how participants perceived filial responsibilities. It not only reflected their 'remembering' of their parents' lives in 'those' years as being full of hardship, framed by the other two discourses (of parental sacrifice and forgetting), but also revealed a value placed on action and practice. Instead of emphasising emotional and spiritual care, participants endeavoured to provide financial and practical care by enabling parents to 'eat and dress well'.

In relation to spirituality, as explained in Chapter 5, most of my participants explicitly indicated that they did not understand the meaning of this word. Even after I tried to explain its meaning and its difference from religiosity (as one participant mistook spirituality for supernatural beliefs), they still either tried to avoid the topic or appeared not to able to understand it. Their care behaviours and anticipations were more focused on practical care—and this was evident not only during the interviews but also from my observations in the hospital setting.

Other aspects of the narratives identified in the analysis were that participants did not explicitly communicate with their parents about their emotions such as love, sorrow, regret, or distress, and this further pointed to the pragmatic focus of their interactions. For example, participants did not verbalise emotions by saying things such as 'I love you' to their parents. They also would not talk about death with their parents as a means of assisting themselves or their parents to reconcile the approaching end-of-life, with cultural and health-related beliefs leading them to refuse to reveal the truth about the illness to the parents. However, this did not mean that they did not communicate with their dying parents. They did not need to say 'I love you' in words but rather expressed their love through practical care and assistance. They refused to tell the truth about the illness to their parents because they thought their silence would provide their parents with more mental strength for their recovery, which is another practical way of showing love and providing care.

As identified in the discussion, this emphasis on action/practice resonated with a pragmatism that is also evident in Chinese philosophies, mainly Confucianism, and in FDA, as discussed in Chapter 4; indeed, Chinese philosophies were significantly focused on practice and action (Liang, 2012; Song, 2008; Wang, 2010), and Foucault's discourse theory also values practice and action as extremely important aspects of discourse (Foucault, 1980).

Complexity of the Discourse of Filial Piety

The complexity of the discourse of filial piety results in part from alterations in terms of migrant peasant workers' social and political status. As discussed in Chapter 9, migrant peasant workers were considered heroic in 'those years'. Since China's economic reform, they have often been depicted as less modern. Indeed, migrant peasant workers are marginalised in the cities in which they work, as articulated by P15 in Chapter 6. Changes in the status of migrant peasant workers also indicate the complexity of migrant peasant workers' discursive formation of culturally embedded values and practices such as filial piety.

A duality in terms of filial piety was detected from my participants' narratives. Filial piety is seen as the predominantly important resource that my participants drew upon to not only make sense of but also enable caring for parents after their diagnosis with cancer. At the same time, the analysis of participants' narratives also revealed that the discourses of filial piety prevented them from asking for help from the government as well as from friends, work colleagues, and relatives. For example, as mentioned in Chapter 6, they could not tell their friends or work colleagues that their parents were dying because of the discursive taboo of talking about death and also for fear that it might result in embarrassment associated with perceptions that they might be hinting that they needed financial assistance.

Change in Discourse of Filial Piety

The concept of change not only relates to the challenges migrant peasant workers who are caring for parents have to face due to urbanisation and their marginalised social status. There have also been many other contextual changes in China, including increasing expectations for high-quality accessible health care and the development of institutional care facilities (Leng et al., 2019). These wider changes have the potential to destabilise the domination of the family care system in China as well as alleviate family care duties. As the Chinese government continues to develop and reform the welfare system, there may be a more promising future for welfare building. Meanwhile, by comparison to their access in 'those years', rural residents have lost access to universal collective social security. From the analysis, it seems there is a discursive 'forgetting' in the political and public discourse.

The embodiment of the concept of change in my participants' comments was their worry that the next generation might not be as filial as them. This worry also indicated their limited trust in the government's promises to build up social welfare. In contemporary Chinese society, despite the Chinese government's expressed intentions to upgrade the current social welfare system, the rural social safety net for rural elders is not comprehensive. The main source of care is still mainly adult children, who often work far away from home. However, factors such as concerns about increasing materialism and self-orientation of the next generation and geographic distance between children and parents led my participants to worry about whether their own children would be filial to them when the time came for them to need such assistance.

Implications and Significance of My Research

My research suggests that techniques of parrhesia (discussed in Chapter 9) may offer some form of resolution to the worries my participants expressed about how eldercare could be sustained in light of the possible diminishment of filial piety in future generations. The first step to the crafting of locally appropriate compromise solutions might be a realisation of the discursive construction of filial piety in 'those years'.

My research fills gaps in the literature, which has heretofore lacked discussion of the construction of filial piety during the GLF and CR. Research to date has also lacked a qualitative focus, and has failed to adequately recognise how migrant peasant workers make sense of their caregiving and how they retain agency in complex contexts, as opposed to merely casting migrant peasant workers as people with a disadvantaged and deprived social status.

A Way Forward for Filial Discourse

A way forward involves tackling such fears about changes to filial piety occurring in the next generation. If we are to take change seriously, we need to understand that change occurs reflexively; a focus on calculating and managing change systematically is bound to result in a doomed attempt to tame change (Nora, 1989). Indeed, the discourse of filial piety is more complex and fluid than can be understood linearly. The identification of parental sacrifice and forgetting discourses revealed complex means via which filial piety is constructed and maintained. If these two mechanisms of (re)constructing filial piety could be made more explicit, and this practice of revealing nuances and deeper understandings could be adopted and enhanced in the next generation, my participants' worries could be mitigated to a great extent. In order for that to occur, something that was 'forgotten' or not provided would have to be 'remembered'.

The Foucauldian concept of parrhesia fits well with this need to remember the forgotten. If my participants and others in similar positions were to remember how their parents' lives were not just full of hardship and sacrifice and how the parental sacrifice discourse was constructed to affect themselves, they might apprehend the possibility that their children would also construct a discourse of parental sacrifice. For example, all of the factors influencing filial piety, such as the personal gain involved in developing a 'good' reputation, the reciprocal benefits of grandchild rearing, and the working through of various forms of emotions, are relevant to current and future familial relationships. Additionally, caregivers could begin to speak out to the government about their needs and expectations, so that the government may know what can be done to improve its policy decisions.

On the government's side, becoming conscious of the identified forgetting discourse creates a possibility for the government to take an opportunity to improve its support system for adult child caregivers of elderly parents, especially those diagnosed with terminal illness. As mentioned in Chapters 3, 8, and 9, it is not just neoliberal reforms that have diminished filial care practice, nor is the government solely responsible for the care challenges that caregivers such as my participants face. The Chinese government has engaged in continuous reforms and attempts to build up a welfare system, albeit the incompleteness of these attempts. If the government could also encourage parrhesia and value more nuanced accounts of the past, it could face criticisms of the GLF and CR, more fully admit to its having discontinued policies on filial piety, and commit to achieving the level of assistance for eldercare promised in the early reform era. Yes, there were policy discrepancies in 'those years'. However, it may be helpful to also recognise the positive aspects and benefits of some policies developed during the GLF and CR as this may enhance continuity with the ongoing social and political reforms on which the Chinese government has embarked in more recent years. For now, the current welfare system is not comprehensive or equitable for rural Chinese. Nonetheless, the Chinese government has shown a will to upgrade the safety net for all older persons and has expressed interest in searching for a more sustainable way to establish a social welfare system in the wake of the crisis of western European socialism that has occurred in recent decades (Mattila & Rapeli, 2018). However, laws such as the 'parent-visiting law' lack practicability. Therefore, there is a need to implement more pragmatic laws and supporting policies.

Research Significance

My research is able to fill in research gaps identified in Chapter 3, to some extent. The two identified discourses of parental sacrifice and forgetting shaped my understanding of the current discursive formation of filial piety in contemporary Chinese society. Instead of solely investigating the care behaviours and patterns of adult children, these two discourses are a result of a deeper discourse analysis, and thereby provide a better understanding of how filial discourse is subjectively (re)constructed and perceived in a changing context in China. These two discourses of filial piety reveal more than just participants' subjective formations of their own care experiences; they also unveil a series of social contexts and transitions of historical periods. In particular, the archaeological and genealogical exploration of filial piety revealed, and began to fill, a gap in the literature on the impact of the GLF and CR on the historical trajectory of filial piety and family caregiving.

As discussed in Chapter 3, there is a lack of qualitative research data in intergenerational care and filial care in the Chinese research arena. My research provides a deep FDA of participants' subjective explanations and narratives. The two discursive mechanisms distilled from the findings, which were identified from the analysis of the qualitative data, may not be able to be generalised to all migrant peasant workers. For example, in this research, most of the participants were recruited at the field hospital. The recruitment method excluded the possibility of recruiting any migrant peasant workers who did not provide care for their ill parents. However, this limitation is inevitable in qualitative research, and its identification can lead to future quantitative and qualitative research. For instance, quantitative research could be done to examine the family care-related concerns of a larger number of migrant peasant workers in China.

The importance of migrant peasant workers as informal caregivers is firmly acknowledged in my research. The low visibility of migrant peasant workers as caregivers in Chinese research was demonstrated in Chapter 3. Migrant peasant workers often are the main source of care for rural elders in China. However, they are facing a lot of challenges in contemporary Chinese society. Therefore, policymakers should consider ways to support their caregiving. My research provides useful data for current and future policymakers, including those who initiated and attempt to implement the recently passed 'parent-visiting law'.

Implications and Recommendations for Policies and Future Research Possibilities

My research identified the pragmatic elements of my participants' narratives and followed up on these elements in theorising about action/practice. In this section, I will follow through on this imperative to theorise for practice by addressing implications and making recommendations for policymakers. Another significant contribution to future research is the theoretical exploration and effort to develop a means of merging Chinese and western methodologies or of localising western methodology in the Chinese context. My research takes steps towards this methodological development by identifying similarities between Foucault's discourse theory and Chinese philosophies that emerged both from the literature and in the analysis of my research data. Additionally, future recommendations for other aspects of research possibilities are also discussed in this section.

Action/Practice and Implications for Future Policies

Action/practice-oriented filial discourse has an extremely important place in current Chinese society (He & van Heugten, 2020). Considering the contextual factors affecting China as a developing country and the fact that the Chinese government has not yet built a comprehensive social care system for older persons, filial care becomes extremely important, as many Chinese scholars have agreed (for example, He & van Heugten, 2020; Liu, 2005). The question in the present remains how policymakers can support and facilitate filial care, especially for people such as my participants (migrant peasant workers).

The criticisms that have been levelled against the newly passed 'parent-visiting law' (2013) have not stopped just at the identification of its unworkability: they have also pointed out its lack of utility as a response to the need to provide for eldercare, as discussed in Chapter 8. As most participants agreed, the educational intent of this law to instil filial morality is 'good' and virtuous. However, participants' observations indicated that the law did not affect them as they were already being filial. They also said that most Chinese people were filial just like them. In other words, according to my participants, this law was not useful or held little purpose for most Chinese people. Needless to say, both the Chinese government and Chinese people have a will to promote filial piety for various reasons. This law does not provide the support and assistance that people such as my participants need; what it does is establish vague criteria for punishment if people do not visit their parents often. If the law is not useful, might there be better approaches? Perhaps the action/practice orientation inherent in Chineseness can help to illuminate a way forward towards a 'solution'.

As indicated from my participants' interviews, since adult children feel reluctant to ask for help, policymakers should endeavour to facilitate filial piety's mediating role to enhance the ways in which filial piety contributes to positive resources, and overcomes the more burdensome implications of filial piety, by formulating and implementing practical and culturally sensitive supporting policies. Services for family caregivers are still widely lacking, although some cities have started to initiate policies for the support of home-based care for elders (PRWeb, 2013). China's recent release of its Temporary Action on Personal Tax Deduction Policy (December 2018), which reduces personal tax if the person has parents over the age of 60 to support, may offer some financial support to caregivers of elderly parents. However, this law is less helpful for migrant workers as many employers do not deduct tax from their earnings and there can therefore be no rebate (Luo, 2018). There is a need for more practical legislation and policies to directly and indirectly support migrant workers as family caregivers, in terms of increasing resources for care available to them. For example, legislation could be put in place to institute provisions for family care-related leave among private companies and factories. Employers might need to be incentivised to apply for such provisions through, for example, providing for reductions in employers' tax if such leaves are granted. Such policies would embody the second element of the conceptual framework, that of action/practice orientedness.

Within China, and outside of China when working with first- and second-generation Chinese immigrants, social services can take better account also of the emotional isolation of family caregivers by, for example, offering culturally sensitive counselling services (undertaken by social workers and counsellors in hospitals) to caregivers and care receivers on dealing with death. This would provide care receivers with an opportunity to confront and deal with their own impending death and may enable caregivers to achieve some emotional closure by being able to say goodbye and express gratitude to their loved one, as well as allowing them to open up to their friends and colleagues for emotional support. However, it is crucial to ensure such services are not imposed on people and that professionals do not unwittingly or deliberately and insensitively force disclosures. The third element of the conceptual framework, parrhesia, is embedded in this discussion of how migrant workers and professionals might balance the importance of attending to cultural imperatives and the need to tackle practical issues and stressors arising from filial care. It is also important to note that issues arising due to divergent cultural practices and deeply held beliefs are difficult to resolve through policies but require relational negotiation. How progress around this can be effectively achieved requires much further examination. Meanwhile, improved knowledge about the importance of filial piety and the different perspectives that may be held by first- and second-generation Chinese immigrants in western countries may go some way towards preventing cross-cultural misunderstanding and distress.

Theoretical Implications

One of the important intentions of my research is to pave the way for the creation of a Chinese methodology for social issues, perhaps borrowing from existing western social theories. As mentioned in Chapter 3, Chinese sociology has failed to develop a Chinese methodology. According to Liu (2014), Chinese modernity has been strongly influenced by the western modernity. However, it also contains its own characteristics and features, and these are embodied in people's everyday practices and perceptions. Social matters and phenomena associated with Chinese modernity need a suitable methodology to lay the foundation for research, which calls for a mutual understanding between the west and China culturally and theoretically.

Within this book's theorisation, filial piety was conceptualised in terms of the similarities between FDA and ancient Chinese philosophies (mainly Confucianism). In order to locate western methodology within the Chinese perspective, I identified three similarities: complexity (and relationality), action orientation, and cultivation of the self. These similarities laid the theoretical foundation for my approach to the research and held important implications for my research findings. According to Wang (2010), Foucault's criticism of western modernity and the uncertainty of his methodological tool for research enable the possibility of achieving a blended methodology in the Chinese context. Additionally, as discussed in Chapter 5, as both an insider and outsider, my reflexive journey between Foucault's theorisation and Chinese traditional theorisation granted me an ability to place myself into the shoes of both theoretical systems and thereby reflexively relate the similarities to my analysis. I highly recommend future researchers to take further steps to develop a Chinese methodology or methodologies, and to search back into ancient roots as well as adopting aspects of western theories to provide a better fit with Chinese modernity. I hope that my research may serve as a solid transition for the realisation of such possibilities in future theoretical and methodological developments.

Future Research into Gender and Spirituality

Filial piety is gendered in its traditional discourse (Gan & Feng, 2020). Ikels (2004) noted that according to Confucian ideals, sons, especially the eldest son, should be mainly responsible for parents' care. The eldest daughter-in-law was seen as the main source for hands-on care for elders in traditional China. Daughters were expected to become caregivers for their husband's parents once they married out of their own family. As discussed in Chapter 6, this gendered discursive content of filial piety is changing. During my fieldwork, I was only able to recruit one daughter-in-law in the hospital, and indeed did not identify any other daughters-in-law in that hospital. The recruited daughter-in-law had her own health conditions and therefore could not take on many care duties. Although some of the male participants still took on the main financial responsibility, several said this was only due to their financial ability. Some participants expressed an opinion that there is no gender difference in terms of providing care for parents but only a difference in terms of one's availability and capability. Despite these expressed views, differences in terms of care were perceptible in the division of labour around specific care tasks. Some participants thought that daughters were more detail-oriented, although the will to care for parents was the same. Gender differences presented in terms of the parent's gender. Daughters attended more with hands-on care if the patient was a mother and sons attended more if the patient was a father, due to the nature of certain tasks such as toileting and changing clothes. The sons were also not as expressive in terms of their emotions as the daughters. Most daughters shared their sorrows and tears during the interview, in contrast to the sons. According to Shi (2009), the gendered aspect of the discourse of filial piety has been changing. Although my research findings appear to support this, I did not have an opportunity to deeply investigate changes in gendered discourses of filial piety. It would be appropriate to examine this issue in future research.

Another possibility for future research is around the question of spirituality. As discussed briefly in this chapter, spirituality was not fully understood by my participants. In my original plan, spirituality was included among topics of interest, because in international intergenerational research, filial piety and end-of-life care are often presumed to be imbued with cultural and spiritual significance (Izuhara, 2010; Zimmer, 2016). Researching discourses of spirituality in China would constitute a large and complex project, one that could potentially be focused on addressing the definition of spirituality in the Chinese context in relation to discourses of filial piety.

Conclusion

To investigate the discourse of filial piety is meaningful for Chinese society today, where family care is still the main source of care for rural elders. An important first step is to acknowledge that it is too simplistic to blame neoliberal market economic reform for the decline of filial practice and perceptions. Unravelling the complexity of filial discourse through migrant peasant workers' interviews revealed mechanisms that can lead to a deeper understanding. Understanding of the mechanisms embedded in discourses of parental sacrifice and forgetting could potentially assuage fears that future generations will not be filial, instead illuminating that they may be differently filial. Acknowledgement of complex discursive practices and some obfuscations may also provide a means of overcoming the relatively low trust that currently exists in relation to the government's capacity to provide a solid social security net for rural families anytime soon (which my participants did not think was the government's responsibility anyway). Parental sacrifice discourse and forgetting discourse could be strengthened on the subjective filial side (through 'new' versions of parental sacrifice such as grandchild rearing, heavy investment in education, and so on) at the same time as they could be deconstructed (through 'telling the truth' about the GLF and CR, for example) at the governmental level. This may support the necessary progression of new governmental policies designed to strengthen the traditional culture of filial piety. Finally, I hope my research will contribute to facilitating future theoretical developments in terms of constructing a methodology that fits in with Chinese modernity.

References

Anonymous. (2013, April 22). *China aged care industry & rare earth industry 2012–2015 new market research report* (2013, July 9). Researchmoz. Retrieved from http://www.prweb.com/releases/2013/4/prweb10655868.htm on October 10, 2019.

Chan, C. L., Ho, A. H., Leung, P. P., Chochinov, H. M., Neimeyer, R. A., Pang, S. M., & Tse, D. M. (2012). The blessings and the curses of filial piety on dignity at the end-of-life: Lived experience of Hong Kong Chinese adult children caregivers. *Journal of Ethnic and Cultural Diversity in Social Work, 21*(4), 277–296. https://doi.org/10.1080/15313204.2012.729177

Cheung, C. K., & Kwan, A.Y.-H. (2009). The erosion of filial piety by modernisation in Chinese cities. *Ageing and Society, 29*(2), 179–198. https://doi.org/10.1017/S0144686X08007836

Cohen, S. A., Cook, S., Kelley, L., Sando, T., & Bell, A. E. (2015). Psychosocial factors of caregiver burden in child caregivers: Results from the new national study of caregiving. *Health and Quality of Life Outcomes, 13*(1), 120. https://doi.org/10.1186/s12955-015-0317-2

Foucault, M. (1980). *Language, counter-memory, practice: Selected essays and interviews*. Blackwell.

Gan, X., & Feng, X. (2020). The diminishment of filial piety or gendered difference: Comparison of filial perceptions between generations from children's perspective 孝道衰落还是儿女有别——子女视角下中青年人养老孝道观的比较研究. *Chinese Youth Research* 中国青年研究 (003), 4–15.

Gruijters, R. J. (2017a). Family care-giving and living arrangements of functionally impaired elders in rural China. *Ageing and Society, 37*(3), 633–647. https://doi.org/10.1017/S0144686X15001397

Gruijters, R. J. (2017b). Intergenerational contact in Chinese families: Structural and cultural explanations. *Journal of Marriage and Family, 79*(3), 758–768. https://doi.org/10.1111/jomf.12390

He, L., & van Heugten, K. (2020). Chinese migrant workers' care experiences: A model of the mediating roles of filial piety. *Qualitative Health Research, 30*(11), 1–13. https://doi.org/10.1177/1049732320925420

Ikels, C. (2004). *Filial piety: Practice and discourse in contemporary East Asia*. Stanford University Press.

Izuhara, M. (2010). *Ageing and intergenerational relations: Family reciprocity from a global perspective*. Policy.

Leng, Y., Liu, W., Xiao, N., Li, Y., & Deng, J. (2019). The impact of policy on the intangible service efficiency of the primary health care institution-based on china's health care reform policy in 2009. *International Journal for Equity in Health, 18*(1), 1–16.

Li, J., Davis, M. P., & Gamier, P. (2011). Palliative medicine: Barriers and developments in mainland China. *Current Oncology Reports, 13*(4), 290–294. https://doi.org/10.1007/s11912-011-0169-9

Liang, D. (2012). *School of Guoxue: The origin of* Guoxue 国学堂:国学溯源. Science Publisher 科学出版社.

Liu, H. (2005). The constructive feature of the pension system in rural China 中国农村养老保障制度建设的阶段性. *Huazhong Technology University Press (Social Science)* 华中科技大学学报: 社会科学版, *19*(1), 72–75. http://skxb.hust.edu.cn/

Liu, Z. (2014). Once upon a time in China: Nationalism, modernity, and cinematic representation. *Frontiers in Literary Studies in China, 8*(4), 532–554.

Luo, Y. (2018). Problems existing in the payment of individual income tax by peasant workers in construction industry 建筑业中农民工缴纳个人所得税存在的问 题. *Modern Economic Information* (22), Article 259. https://doi.org/10.3969/j.issn.1001-828X.2018.33.205

Mattila, M., & Rapeli, L. (2018). Just sick of it? Health and political trust in western Europe. *European Journal of Political Research, 57*(1), 25–33.

Nora, P. (1989). Between memory and history: Les lieux de mémoire. *Representations, 26*, 7–24. http://www.representations.org/

Shi, L. (2009). 'Little quilted vests to warm parents' hearts': Redefining the gendered practice of filial piety in rural north-eastern China. *The China Quarterly, 198*(198), 348–363. https://doi.org/10.1017/S0305741009000344

Song, Z. (2008). *Chinese traditional philosophic discussion* 中国传统哲学通. People's University of China Press.

Wang, D. (2010). *The fall of humanity* 人类的没落. Xianxi People's Publisher.

Yang, Y. (2009). An investigation of aged care in migrant peasant worker families—A case study of several towns of Yibing city in Sichuan province 农民

工家庭的养老状况调查——四川省宜宾县部分乡镇的实证研究. *Decision and Information Quarterly* 决策与信息旬刊 (11), 188–189. http://www.jcyxx.com/

Zhang, T. (2016). *Speed up legislation of ethnic and folk traditional culture*. http://www.npc.gov.cn/npc/dbdhhy/12_4/2016-03/13/content_1981743.htm

Zhou, A. (2011). A discussion of social security for 'empty nest' rural elders 浅谈中国农村"空巢"家庭的养老保障问题. *China Agricultural Studies* 中国农学通报, *27*(14), 151–156. http://www.casb.org.cn/casb/ch/index.aspx

Zhu, J. (2019). *Suicidal perceptions and reasons among rural elders in Shandong province* 山东省农村老年人自杀意念及其影响因素研究 (Doctoral dissertation). Shandong University.

Zhu, L. (2001). Collective discrimination and bias: The conflicting interaction between migrant peasant workers and urban residents 群体性偏见与歧视--农民工与市民的磨擦性互动. *Jianghai Academic Periodical* 江海学刊 (6), 48–53. http://www.jhxk.cn/CN/volumn/home.shtml

Zimmer, Z. (2016). *Global ageing in the twenty-first century: Challenges, opportunities and implications*. Routledge.

The manufacturer's authorised representative in the EU is Springer
Nature Customer Service Centre GmbH, Europaplatz 3, 69115 Heidelberg,
Germany. If you have any concerns regarding our products, please
contact ProductSafety@springernature.com

Printed and bound by CPI Group (UK) Ltd, Croydon, CR0 4YY

30/09/2026

02225455-0012